Duties of a Doctor

Patients must be able to trust doctors with their lives and well-being. To justify that trust, we as a profession have a duty to maintain a good standard of practice and care, and to show respect for human life. In particular as a doctor you must:

- make the care of your patient your first concern;
- treat every patient politely and considerately·
- respect patients' dignity and privacy·
- listen to patients and resp~
- give patients informa
- respect the rights of μ about their care;
- keep your professional k ~o date;
- recognize the limits of you ~ competence;
- be honest and trustworthy;
- respect and protect confidential information;
- make sure that your personal beliefs do not prejudice your patients' care;
- act quickly to protect patients from risk if you have good reason to believe that you or a colleague may not be fit to practise;
- avoid abusing your position as a doctor; and
- work with colleagues in the ways that best serve patients' interests.

In all these matters you must never discriminate unfairly against your patients or colleagues. And you must always be prepared to justify your actions to them.

Duties of a Doctor is reproduced with kind permission of the General Medical Council.

Second Edition

CRASH COURSE

Foundation Doctor's Guide
TO **Medicine**
AND **Surgery**

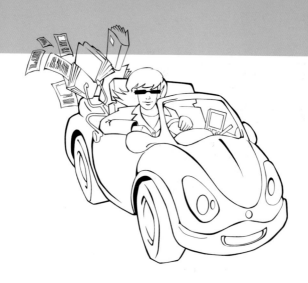

Commissioning Editor: Alison Taylor
Development Editor: Kim Benson
Project Manager: Christine Johnston
Design: Stewart Larking
Illustration Manager/Illustrator: Merlyn Harvey

Second Edition

CRASH COURSE

Foundation Doctor's Guide TO Medicine AND Surgery

Miles Witham BM BCh MRCP(UK)
Clinical Lecturer in Ageing and Health,
Section of Ageing and Health, Ninewells Hospital and
Royal Victoria Hospital, Dundee, UK

Paramjit Jeetley MB ChB MRCP(UK)
Cardiology SpR, Bristol Royal Infirmary, Bristol, UK

Emily Morton MB ChB
F2 House Officer, Ninewells Hospital, Dundee, UK

MOSBY

ELSEVIER

Edinburgh · London · New York · Oxford · Philadelphia · St Louis · Sydney · Toronto 2008

MOSBY
ELSEVIER

First edition 2004
Reprinted 2005
Second edition 2008

ISBN 978-0-7234-3440-5

British Library Cataloguing in Publication Data
A catalogue record for this book is available from the British Library.

Library of Congress Cataloging in Publication Data
A catalog record for this book is available from the Library of Congress.

Note

Knowledge and best practice in this field are constantly changing. As new research and experience broaden our knowledge, changes in practice, treatment and drug therapy may become necessary or appropriate. Readers are advised to check the most current information provided (i) on procedures featured or (ii) by the manufacturer of each product to be administered, to verify the recommended dose or formula, the method and duration of administration, and contraindications. It is the responsibility of the practitioner, relying on their own experience and knowledge of the patient, to make diagnoses, to determine dosages and the best treatment for each individual patient, and to take all appropriate safety precautions. To the fullest extent of the law, neither the Publisher nor the Authors assumes any liability for any injury and/or damage to persons or property arising out or related to any use of the material contained in this book.

The Publisher

ELSEVIER your source for books, journals and multimedia in the health sciences
www.elsevierhealth.com

Working together to grow libraries in developing countries
www.elsevier.com | www.bookaid.org | www.sabre.org

 ELSEVIER   BOOK AID International   Sabre Foundation

The publisher's policy is to use paper manufactured from sustainable forests

Printed in China

Contents

Congratulations – you made it through medical school! You've celebrated your results, changed the name on your credit cards, said farewell to many of your friends and hopefully managed to enjoy a few weeks of relaxation before you begin your first job.

That of course, is the tricky part – the thought of starting work as a doctor can be very daunting, especially as it often involves moving to an unfamiliar hospital in a new town.

This book can help. Like all Crash Course titles, it is designed to be complete, clear and concise – the authors have carefully excluded superfluous material that you are unlikely to need in an average working week, leaving the essential information you will want to refer to every day. White coats are *so* last century – so we have packed all this information into a compact, splash-resistant volume that will fit in your pocket, bag, or work folder. This Second Edition of the title has been specifically updated for the new Foundation Year 1 posts that you will be starting, as well as including more general updates to account for changes in pharmacology and best practice guidelines.

The guide begins with the basic information you need to get started (including what to bring with you on your first day) and then moves on to cover the common practical tasks that you will be performing every day as a Foundation Year 1 doctor. These are explained in a logical step-by-step manner using clear diagrams. Common pitfalls are highlighted to help you avoid them. Next, the book covers the important medical and surgical emergencies and provides simple diagnostic criteria followed by a list explaining what you should do when you are first on the scene. Finally, it offers an approach to the common medical and surgical presentations, interpretation of common investigations, and clinical examination.

Above all, do not panic! Your first few months as a doctor may occasionally be terrifying, will often be tiring and will certainly be challenging, but they will also be among the most rewarding of your career. There is nothing quite like the realisation, a few days or weeks into the job, that you *can* do it. This, together with the opportunities to make new friends, learn new skills and finally put your training into action, can make your years as a foundation doctor truly exhilarating and enjoyable.

I wish you the best of luck in your future careers.

Dr Dan Horton-Szar

The world of medical training moves on, and to reflect these changes, a new edition of this Crash Course guide is required. The traditional House Officer year is now a 2-year Foundation programme with an expanded syllabus and exposure to many more specialities. Fundamentally, however, the challenges remain the same as they always have been: working in new environments; collaborating with new colleagues and facing up to new clinical responsibilities. All of these are terrifying and thrilling in equal measure, though the balance tends to favour the former initially!

Our aim is that this new edition of our 'survival guide' continues to provide the support and advice of its predecessor. To reflect the brave new world, there is a new chapter on the Foundation years, as well as updated chapters on medical and surgical emergencies to incorporate current guidelines, as well as an enhanced chapter on ECG interpretation. As we have said previously, the information provided here is almost certainly not new, but merely a reminder of knowledge that is already there but just needs a little prompt in times of stress.

We hope that this book will help you do more than survive the occasional stormy voyage through your Foundation years. Medicine is an enjoyable and stimulating career, and though life can be tough at times, the rewards are immense. It is important to keep things in perspective and if at all possible . . . enjoy the ride!

Miles Witham
Paramjit Jeetley
Emily Morton

Our immense thanks are due to Mr Bill Neary, SpR in General Surgery, Bristol Royal Infirmary for his significant contribution to the surgical chapters.

As always, thanks to both Helen and Justine for their patience as well as to Kim for her prompt and efficient editing.

Acknowledgements

The basics

The basics

Your first day

Your first day at work will be a blur of new places, new faces, induction lectures and paperwork. You will be given an enormous amount of information and the trick is to prioritize – don't try to remember everything you are told.

To take with you on the first day:

- GMC certificate • Medical records, including hepatitis B status • Bank details
- A4 size folder or notebook • Black pens • Stethoscope • Tourniquet • Pen torch • Money • This book

---

You might not need all of the above if the hospital has seen your details beforehand. So what is important? We suggest the following things should be your priorities:

Your contract. Many hospitals are very tardy when it comes to giving you a contract. Demand one on the first day and make sure that you read it carefully. If you don't like what you see (e.g. pay banding for overtime), don't sign it – talk to your BMA representative first.

Your timetable and rota. Find out what occurs when, and what is expected of you. The best thing to do is to talk to your predecessor in the job; you might have the opportunity of shadowing them for a day or two before starting the job yourself. Find out when you are on call.

Computers. Find out how to work the ward computers and apply for a password on the first day. Passwords often take several days to be allocated and until you have one you will find accessing test results (and ordering tests in some hospitals) very difficult.

Lists. Get a list of useful phone numbers and bleeps, including labs and radiology.

Payroll. If you haven't signed a payroll form, sign it on your first day. If you don't give your details to payroll, you don't get paid – and payroll might then not be able to pay you the first month.

Occupational health. If you haven't visited occupational health before starting the job, arrange to see them – preferably within the first day or two. This is particularly important if you haven't got a current hepatitis B status – you cannot undertake invasive procedures without confirmation of hepatitis B immune status.

Holidays. Sit down with your colleagues in the first couple of days and decide when you all want to take holidays. It is much better to get this sorted out early on in the job; if you wait until halfway through the post, you won't get to take all of your holiday entitlement.

Living arrangements. Find out where you are staying as soon as you arrive at the hospital. Find out where you sleep when on call, where to get food, where the supermarket is and where the mess is.

Your team and your patients. When you have sorted out the list above, go and find your team and your patients. Introduce yourself to the nurses on your home ward and get familiarized with where everything is. If you are lucky, you will have either spent time on the ward as a medical student or shadowed the previous foundation doctor. Someone from the team should be able to hand over your bleep as well.

That is quite enough for a first day. Pensions, pharmacy information, fire lectures and other paraphernalia can wait, and be dealt with over the next few days.

Don't worry about taking a lot of paper and books around with you; you will be weighed down with too much kit and things will get lost. An A4 folder or hardbound A4 notebook is ideal for storing spare forms, patient lists, timetables, etc. and is an ideal place for your list of jobs to do. You can decide either to take tools such as a tendon hammer and ophthalmoscope with you (but see above) or, if you need to do a neurological exam, risk having to hunt for the equipment.

What to write

General points

Note-writing is one of those tasks that is perceived to be very easy but is often done exceptionally badly. The reason for this is that it is often not taught at medical school and, as a foundation doctor, you are expected to know what to write from your first day. There are several reasons to ensure that notes are kept well:

- They provide a clear and accurate account of the patient's management – if it's not written, it was not done.
- They allow communication to others of what was said and done.
- They are a legal document and can be used in court.
- They provide information for audit and research.
- There are some universal features that apply to note-making regardless of specialty or seniority:
  - Legibility: 'doctors' handwriting' is thankfully now becoming a myth, although there are still examples around. You must make your writing legible. If it is not, and what you have written is misunderstood, you will not get the benefit of the doubt. You are now also required to write in black at all times, as this is much clearer if the notes are photocopied.
  - Patient identification: every new sheet of paper in the notes should have at least three points of identification on it: (i) patient's name (surname and forename); (ii) patient's date of birth; and (iii) patient's hospital number. If the hospital number is unavailable, use the first line of the patient's address.
  - Date and time: every entry made in the notes must be dated (including the year – patients do return) and preferably timed. Timing is especially important when patients are acutely unwell or when there is a lot of activity, e.g. postoperatively.
  - Abbreviations: difficult to avoid but try to just use conventional ones, e.g. FBC and COPD, and write others out.
  - Signature: you must sign every entry you make in a set of notes. If your signature is illegible, then print your name beneath so it is clear who you are.

Clerking a patient

The basic structure of any clerking is the same. How much detail there is in each section is variable, but the structure should be:

- patient details
- date and time of entry
- method of referral
- history
- examination
- impression
- investigations
- plan
- signature and bleep number

METHOD OF REFERRAL

Whether the admission was as an emergency or elective/routine, and by whom the referral was made, e.g. GP or A&E.

HISTORY

Taking a history and documenting it is an art that you will develop throughout your medical career. The key is simplicity and clarity of thought. If your thoughts are a mess, this is reflected in your note-making.

If no history is available, e.g. if the patient is confused or has a reduced level of consciousness, you should try and obtain a history from other sources, e.g. relatives, nursing home, etc.

Presenting complaint (PC) This is usually one word – usually the patient's own, e.g. cough or breathlessness. Sometimes there can be two or three, e.g. 1. palpitations, 2. chest pain.

History of presenting complaint (HPC) This expands on the presenting complaint or complaints. An example is if the presenting complaint is 'Pain', go on to describe the onset of pain. When discussing times, try to use relative values such as '3 h ago' or '2 days ago' as opposed to 'yesterday'.

The history is where the bulk of your clerking relevant to that admission will be. It is therefore acceptable to put in entries that will also be in other categories, such as past medical history, social history or medication.

Medication Documentation of the patient's drugs and their doses on admission is important because this will be what you base your prescription chart on. You will need to phone the patient's GP, or ask a relative to bring in any drugs a patient is taking, if the patient has not brought them to hospital or is unsure what they are. The key to the diagnosis could lie in what the patient is (or is not) taking.

Allergies Allergies to drugs should always be asked about; omitting to do this is medicolegally indefensible.

Social history This section is often overlooked but might be very relevant to the patient's admission, particularly in older people. In this population it is important to know the level of independence and how much the patient can do normally, e.g. wash, dress, shop. A decrease in the level of function in a short time might be the only feature in the history leading to the admission, and might have an organic cause, e.g. infection.

Review of systems This is a brief review of all systems not already covered by the main part of the history. This is there for completeness and to check you haven't missed any clinically relevant parts of the history.

EXAMINATION

Documentation of a clinical examination again is tailored to your history. Whereas a detailed neurological examination is mandatory for a patient presenting with a stroke, it is less relevant for a patient presenting for elective hernia repair. Nevertheless, a competent efficient examination of the major systems (CVS, respiratory, abdominal and nervous) should lead to concise notes that reflect your clinical findings. These should always include vital signs such as pulse and blood pressure – this demonstrates that you have seen the relevant measurements and acknowledged them.

A note about CNS examination

Assessing power and reflexes involves a mysterious combination of fractions and crosses. Here is an explanation:

Grading of power

5/5	Normal
4/5	Slightly reduced
3/5	Able to overcome gravity, i.e. able to lift off bed
2/5	Unable to overcome gravity i.e. unable to lift off bed but can maintain if raised
1/5	Slight movement; muscle twitch only
0/5	No movement

Grading of reflexes

+++	Exaggerated
++	Normal
+	Present with reinforcement
+/−	Equivocal
−	Absent

IMPRESSION

This is what you think is going on with your patient. Everything that follows is tailored to prove or disprove your theory. It is not a diagnosis yet and no-one is going to shoot you if your impression is wrong.

INVESTIGATIONS

Although some of the investigations are 'routine', they are there so you can start proving your impression. For example, if you have a patient who presents with left-sided pleuritic chest pain and cough, your clinical impression might be that of pneumonia. You might also want to exclude a pneumothorax and a pulmonary embolism. The investigation list might therefore read something like Fig. 1.

Investigations

FBC
U + Es
Glucose
Cardiac enzymes
CRP

ECG
CXR
ABGs
Consider V/Q scan

Fig. 1 Sample investigations list for a patient who presents with left-sided pleuritic chest pain and cough.

PLAN

Your plan consists of two things:

1. your immediate management plan
2. your plan for the next 24–48 hours

This could be as simple as admitting the patient and reviewing the results of the tests with your seniors, or as complicated as administration of drugs and practical procedures. Try to avoid simply writing 'senior review' – if the patient is so sick your senior needs to review immediately you will not get a chance to write any notes; if you do have time, then you also have time to think about what you want to do. For example, Fig. 2 might apply to a patient with pleuritic chest pain.

An example of a clerking is given in Fig. 3.

Progress notes and ward rounds

After you have clerked the patient, you will go on ward rounds, mostly under the supervision of a more senior doctor, who will quite often expect you to write in the notes as you go. You must therefore be aware of what is going on with the patients' management, and to do this you must be attentive to what is going on. If you do not understand – ask. This is particularly important on the post-take ward round, where the working diagnosis is decided. If you understand what is going on at this stage, not only will you learn how to manage patients for yourself in the future, but you will be able to write down the plan for the patient with confidence.

Progress notes broadly fall into the same categories as clerking notes:

- date and time
- who is leading the ward round
- history
- examination
- investigations
- plan
- signature

The difference is that you might write just one line for each. The emphasis is that each set of notes will follow on, so the reader who has never met the patient knows

Plan
Oxygen 40%
Co-Dydramol   QDS
R/V with result of CXR and ABGs
If fever, do blood and sputum cultures
Consider antibiotics
R/V SHO

Fig. 2 Example of a plan for a patient with pleuritic chest pain.

John Smith
H1234567
12/3/1930

7.2.2003
23^{00}

E/A via A&E
72-yr-old man

PC Chest pain

HPC Gradually worsening chest pain this week
Commenced at 5/7 ago
Describes as left-sided, sharp pain
No radiation
Worse on inspiration
Settled in ambulance with O_2

Known angina but not similar to
previous angina pains

CABG 1998 Mild CVA post surgery
residual left-sided
weakness
No angina since then
Walks with stick
good exercise
tolerance

Risk factors IHD: Hypertension
↑Chol
Ex-smoker –
10/day for >20 years
°DM °FHx

Meds Aspirin 75 mg OD
Clopidogrel 75 mg OD
Atenolol 50 mg OD
Simvastatin 20 mg OD

PMH °Epil / °Asthma/
COPD/ °TB/ °Jaund
Nil else of note

SHx Independent
Lives with wife
Alcohol : 6U/week

RoS OA back and hips pain on
climbing hills. Nil else of note

Fig. 3 An example of a clerking.

O/E

Comfortable
Temp 37.2

CVS: *Pulse 84 reg*
           BP 150/70
           HS I + II + systolic murmur, loudest at apex
           JVP not elevated
           Apex undisplaced
           No carotid bruits
           Peripheral pulses all present

Resp: *RR = 20*   *Sats 95% on air*
           Trachea central
           AE Good bilaterally
           PN Resonant bilaterally
           BS Vesicular R + L
           Insp crackles L base

Abdo: *Soft non tender*
           No liver/spleen/kidneys palpable
           No masses palpable
           BS Normal
           PR Not performed

CNS: *Normal eye movements*
           No diplopia/nystagmus
           No facial asymmetry
           II XII otherwise intact

	Right	Left
Arms		
Tone	*Normal*	↑
Power	*Normal*	4/5
Legs		
Tone	*Normal*	↑
Power	*Normal*	4/5
Reflexes		
Biceps	++	+++
Triceps	++	+++
Supinator	++	+++
Knees	++	+++
Ankles	++	+++
Planters	↓	↑

Normal proprioception
Gait not assessed

Fig. 3 Cont'd.

8.2.03 PTWR Dr B
08⁴⁵

Pleuritic Left-sided pleuritic chest pain for 1/52.
Assoc^d cough.
No sputum.
Temp 38 this am. Sats 100% on 40% O_2
   BP 140/70 Pulse 80
Chest : Crackles, left base
CXR : L basal shadowing   prob consolidation
       No pneumothorax seen
WCC↑
ECG and cardiac enzymes   N

Imp : Left basal pneumonia

Plan

      Continue on O_2 and monitor sats
      Blood and sputum cultures
      PO Amoxicillin 500 mg TDS
      Not for V/Q   Unlikely to be PE   A Jones 123
                                   F1 to Dr B

9.2.03 WR F2
09³⁰

Pt feels much better. Pain settled.
O/E   Afebrile since yesterday pm
      Chest   odd crackle, left base

Plan: WCC mane
     Mobilize
     Check WCC mane   if OK and pt well, home tom
     Chase blood cultures
            Will need CXR and O/P in 6/52
                              A Jones 123
                              F1 ABC

Fig. 4 Sample progress notes for a patient with pleuritic chest pain.

what your plan is and why you are doing the tests you are. Fig. 4 gives an example for our patient with pleuritic chest pain.

An alternative scheme is 'SOAP':

- Subjective (i.e. how the patient feels)
- Objective (examination findings)
- Assessment (diagnosis, how things are progressing)
- Plan

Night working

Part of the job involves working in the evenings and at night. At this time, when you might be the only doctor awake in your specialty, it is even more important to document clearly the date and time you reviewed a particular patient. The patient is

```
10.2.03        Ward Cover F1
10.30pm        Asked to review patient
Smith

               Patient c/o more chest pain
               O/E remains afebrile
               Crackles left base
               Tender++ over left lower ribs

   Imp         Musculoskeletal pain
   Plan        ↑analgesia to co-Dydramol            QDS
                                          A Smith 456
```

Fig. 5 Sample notes made while on night duty.

quite often not managed by your team in these situations and so it is important to document who you are – writing your surname at the top of your entry as well as signing your notes is a good way of ensuring this (Fig. 5).

Notes of conversations

In your day-to-day life, you will communicate with others regarding the management of patients. The range of people you will deal with is vast, from other healthcare professionals (doctors, nurses, physiotherapists, occupational therapists and social workers) to patients' relatives. If any of these have an impact on your patients' management, it should be documented so a clear record of events is recorded. This is particularly important if any facts are disputed at a later date.

In all of these situations it is important to document when you had a conversation, and with whom. If a conversation with relatives and the patient takes place, note exactly who was present, e.g. 'Discussion with patient and family – daughter (Mrs E Smith) present'.

When you talk to other healthcare professionals, particularly outside your specialty, then their names should be taken so that it is clear with whom the patient was discussed: 'D/w Mr Shah, Surgical Reg on call' with a time documented is better than 'D/w Surgical Reg'. This is particularly important at night, when you might be required to wake someone for advice and their recollection might not be as good as yours in the morning. Precisely document the issues raised in a conversation, particularly if discussing issues with relatives or involving consent.

Old notes and summaries

Quite often you will admit patients who have had several hospital admissions and are well known to the hospital. In this situation, obtaining the old notes is invaluable because they can provide you with another source of information to corroborate your patient's history, particularly if this is unreliable. Secretaries and ward clerks are useful allies in this respect and often find the means of retrieving these sometimes-elusive items for you.

Unfortunately, on arrival, old notes couldn't look more different from the important medicolegal documents they are supposed to be. However, taking the time to sift through the notes and summarizing the patient's history can be extremely useful and most senior doctors will do this routinely to get a handle on a patient's condition. Doing this will help improve your knowledge of the patient's history. Your summary is just that – it need not be an essay – but a list of important milestones in a patient's history can sometimes reveal glaring omissions, which could earn you valuable points on a consultant ward round, not to mention improving the care of your patient.

Filling in forms

One of the mundane tasks of any foundation doctor is form filling. This seemingly menial task has often been felt to be beneath doctors, a task that should be delegated to secretaries or ward clerks. Although it is true that some of it is fairly mundane, only someone with adequate medical knowledge will know which test is indicated and what question they would like answered. As a result, correct form filling is still an essential skill.

Although forms vary from Trust to Trust, the basics are similar:

- Three forms of identification are usually needed: patient name, date of birth and hospital number (or address).
- The patient's location, e.g. ward or outpatients.
- Your name and bleep number.
- Your signature.

If any of these are not present, the request for bloods or investigations will be sent back to you. You will have wasted their time and your own.

Blood forms These are by far the most common forms you will fill in. You should make absolutely sure that the patient's details are correct, particularly when ordering blood products. The section marked 'Clinical Details' should also be filled in – this can be as brief as 'On ACE inhibitor' if you are checking some U+Es on a patient, to more complex details for rarer tests (Fig. 6). If the test is urgent, mark it so on the form and phone the lab to let them know that the sample is on its way.

X-ray forms Although patient details are as important on radiology request forms as they are on blood forms, the clinical details section of this form is absolutely vital. Whatever investigation is requested, remember that the radiologists will not know the patient as well as you do. In fact, the only clinical information the radiologists will have about the patient is what you write in this section – if you give them rubbish, you will get rubbish back in the report. Radiologists need this section to

St Somewhere's Hospital Trust combined investigation form		
Patient name	*A Smith*	ID / DoB	*251041 0104*
Address		GP	*Dr S Jones*
Consultant	*Dr Hart*	Ward:	*15*
Tests requested		Clinical details	
FBC, U+Es, LFTs, CK, TFTs		*Chest pain ? MI. Hypothyroid on thyroxine. Iron deficiency anaemia*	
Signature *D A Kilgannon* Grade *F1*	Date *11/2/03*		Bleep no. *123*

Fig. 6 Example of a completed investigation form for blood tests.

understand what information you hope to gain by performing the investigation. If you do not ask a specific question or do not give the appropriate details, the investigation and subsequent report will not be targeted to your needs.

Your clinical details need not be an essay – just a summary of the patient's clinical state and the question that needs to be answered. Again, knowledge of the patient's working diagnosis is crucial to do this properly, so when you request a test make sure you understand what is going on. It is far harder to explain the patient's state to someone else if you do not know it yourself. So:

- if requesting a chest X-ray, write: 'SOB, cough, smoker 30/day ?infection ?underlying malignancy'

- or if you are requesting a CT of the brain for a patient who has had a stroke, write: 'Left-sided weakness leg and arm. Dysarthria. Stroke – exclude haemorrhage'

Some departments require you to discuss anything but a simple X-ray with one of the radiologists. Don't be scared. In your first weeks this task might seem intimidating – the key is knowing why the test has been requested so that you are prepared if you are confronted with questions.

Fig. 7 shows a sample X-ray form.

Drug charts

Prescribing drugs is an important job that needs to be done accurately. Again, the forms vary between hospitals but the basic layout is consistent. Patient details are found on the front page, together with a section for drug allergies. Both of these sections should be filled in accurately (patient's name, ward, hospital number, etc.).

PRESCRIBING

To prescribe any drug, certain elements should be present:

- Patient details.
- Name of the drug: try to use generic names, not trade names, e.g. metoclopramide not Maxalon. Always prescribe in capitals so there is no doubt as to what you are prescribing.

St Somewhere's Hospital Trust radiology request form

Patient name	*A Smith*	ID / DoB	*251041 0104*
Address		GP	*Dr S Jones*
Consultant	*Dr Hart*	Ward: *15*	
Tests requested		Clinical details	
CXR		*Chest pain ? MI. Breathless at rest, fine crackles at both bases ? Pulmonary oedema*	
Signature *D A Kilgannon* Grade *F1*	Date	*17/2/03*	Bleep no. *123*

Fig. 7 Sample X-ray form.

- Dose of drug: make sure you know this and that it is written clearly. Make the units clear – g or mg or μg.
- Method of delivery: PO (oral), IM (intramuscular), IV (intravenous), SC (subcutaneous), NG (via nasogastric tube). Some hospitals require you to write abbreviations out in full.
- Frequency of administration: OD (once daily), BD (twice daily), TDS (three times a day), QDS (four times a day), prn (as required). Some hospitals discourage the use of Latin abbreviations.
- Times of administration: there are set times for drug rounds on a ward but stating the times for drug administration is important, particularly for single doses or once daily drugs.
- Date of prescription: give the date that the drug was first prescribed during the admissions, not the date you rewrote the drug chart.
- Your signature: no drug can be administered without this.

Other details, such as for how long a drug is prescribed (e.g. for antibiotics), might also be required.

DIFFERENT TYPES OF DRUG CHART

There are usually three ways of prescribing drugs: as one-off doses, as regular doses or on an 'as-required basis'. As a result, there are three sections on a drug chart for all of these.

- 'One-off' doses are usually prescribed on the front of the chart. This is for single doses of medication prescribed in emergencies, when only a single dose of a particular drug is required, or when the dose changes after each administration. Here times should be documented in 24-hour clock, or as 'stat' (immediate) doses (Fig. 8).
- Regular medications are prescribed inside and comprise the bulk of the chart. Again, be clear about times and what you are prescribing (Fig. 9).
- The as-required medication section is important for minor prescribing such as analgesia and antiemetics. Always prescribe a maximum dose to prevent overdosing (Fig. 10).

When amending a drug chart, cross-out the entry clearly and rewrite the prescription. Multiple crossings out on one entry lead to errors in dispensing.

ANTICOAGULATION PRESCRIBING

Most drug charts have a separate section for prescribing unfractionated heparin and warfarin. As the dose might change frequently, there is usually a section where you

Once only medications						
Date	Medication	Dose	Route	Time	Signature	Given
29/2/03	FUROSEMIDE	80 mg	PO	STAT	A Smith	10^{20}
29/2/03	ASPIRIN	300 mg	PO	STAT	A Smith	10^{22}

Fig. 8 Example of a one-off (once only) drug chart.

	Regular medication						
Medication *ASPIRIN*	**Dose**		Date Time	1	2	3	4
			0600				
	75 mg		0800				
			1000				
	Freq *OD*	**Route** *PO*	1200				
			1400				
			1800				
Signature A Smith	**Start** *1.2.03*	**Stop**	2000				
			2200				
			2400				
Medication *FUROSEMIDE*	**Dose**		0600				
			0800				
	80 mg		1000				
	Freq *BD*	**Route** *PO*	1200				
			1400				
			1800				
Signature A Smith	**Start** *1.2.03*	**Stop**	2000				
			2200				
			2400				
Medication *SALBUTAMOL via volumatic*	**Dose** *2 puffs*		0600				
			0800				
			1000				
	Freq *QDS*	**Route** *Inh*	1200				
			1400				
			1800				
Signature A Smith	**Start** *1.2.03*	**Stop**	2000				
			2200				
			2400				

Fig. 9 Example of a drug chart for regular medications.

	As-required medication						
Medication *PARACETAMOL*	**Dose** *500 mg 1 g*		Date Time	1	2	3	4
	Max Freq *QDS*	**Route** *PO*					
Signature A Smith	**Start** *1.2.03*	**Stop**					

Fig. 10 As-required drug chart.

can write the INR and prescribe the appropriate dose for that day. Make sure that you do this every day to avoid your on-call colleagues having to prescribe for you.

FLUID CHARTS

Prescribing intravenous fluids is usually done on a separate fluid chart. These include prescriptions for blood products, such as blood, fresh-frozen plasma and platelets. Again, patient details must be correct with three points of identification (see above).

Conventional fluids (crystalloids) including normal saline (0.9% NaCl solution) or 5% dextrose solution, are available in 100-mL to 1-L bags. These are used for hydrating patients who require fluids and are unable to take adequate amounts by mouth, e.g. they are septic, or nil-by-mouth pre- or postoperative patients. Fluids are usually given over 6–8 h, but can be given more quickly. Caution should be used when prescribing fluids to patients with heart failure or in the elderly – there is the risk of the patient developing pulmonary oedema if fluids are given too quickly. If you are in any doubt, call your senior.

Sometimes, additives are given to the normal crystalloid preparations, e.g. potassium, to replace losses. Be careful with these prescriptions and monitor U+Es closely. Potassium is a dangerous drug and needs close monitoring.

Bags of fluid are also used to dilute drugs that are then infused over a period up to 24 h. Examples include amiodarone and aminophylline – make sure you are certain of the infusion rates and prescribe the correct dose for that volume of fluid, e.g. the slow phase loading dose for amiodarone IV is 900 mg infused over 23 h. It is therefore diluted into 1 L normal saline and the total infused for 23 h (Fig. 11).

Colloids are fluids given when resuscitating patients, e.g. in septic shock and hypovolaemia. They remain in the circulation longer than crystalloids and come in 500-mL bags that, ideally, are given through large peripheral cannulas. They can be infused very rapidly (squeezed in over 2–3 min) or given over 20–30 min.

Blood products must be prescribed meticulously – the consequences of the wrong person receiving a transfusion can be catastrophic and medicolegally indefensible.

Blood or packed red cells are usually given over around 4 h. In the elderly, or in patients with heart failure, they can be given over 6 h. You might also need to prescribe a small dose of furosemide (usually 20 mg given orally) to prevent excess fluid accumulation if the patient is not hypovolaemic and is prone to heart failure; this is often the case in elderly patients. Platelets and FFP are given over 20–30 min.

SLIDING SCALES

Insulin sliding scales prescriptions vary from hospital to hospital but most places use an intravenous method, changing the infusion of insulin according to the patient's

Fluid prescription for amiodarone					
Fluid and volume	Additive	Infusion rate	Signature	Start	Stop
0.9% saline 1L	AMIODARONE 900 mg	23 hours	A Smith	13⁰⁵	

Fig. 11 Fluid prescription chart for a maintenance dose of amiodarone.

Fluid prescription for insulin					
Fluid and volume	Additive	Infusion rate	Signature	Start	Stop
0.9% saline 50 mL	50 U ACTRAPID	As per sliding scale	A Smith	16²⁰	
BM	Rate of infusion				
> 17 11 –17	6 mL/h 4 mL/h		A Smith		
7 –11 4 –7	2 mL/h 1 mL/h				
3 < 4	0.5 mL/h				

Fig. 12 Fluid prescription sheet for an insulin sliding scale.

blood glucose. Use a fluid prescription sheet when prescribing an intravenous sliding scale. Insulin is usually given as an infusion of a short-acting insulin, e.g. Actrapid in an equal amount of fluid; this gives easy correlation between the infusion rate and the amount of insulin given, i.e. 1 mL/h of infusion is 1 unit/h of insulin (Fig. 12).

Fig. 12 is a slightly complex example, with lots of dose changes, but simpler sliding scales can be used just as effectively, e.g. BM > 10 infusion rate 6 mL/h or BM < 10 infusion rate 3 mL/h.

Remember, fluids are usually prescribed together with a sliding scale. Insulin also lowers potassium in the blood so monitor U+Es in anyone on an IV sliding scale (see 'Diabetic ketoacidosis', p. 105).

Death certification

People die in hospitals. When they do, they create a mass of paperwork that must be filled in correctly to prevent any delay in what is already a difficult time for relatives.

The first stage is to declare the patient dead. Many, many stories are told of doctors declaring a patient dead, only for the patient to 'come back to life', causing embarrassment all round.

Deaths in hospital are either expected or after a failed resuscitation at cardiac arrest. In the post-arrest situation, do not certify immediately but leave the room and write up your notes. Return after a few minutes and examine the body at that stage. If you are called to an expected death, go to the ward promptly so the patient's relatives can be called and the body then removed to the mortuary.

Examination of the patient should involve:

- checking the response to a painful stimulus
- checking the major pulse – carotid or femoral – for 60 s
- listening for heart sounds
- watching and listening for breath sounds for at least 3 min
- checking pupil reaction to light

17

If all of these are negative then fully document the time of death, the time you certified the patient, your findings confirming death and sign your entry.

DEATH CERTIFICATES

The death certificate is a legal document and as a result must be filled in correctly, not least because bereaved relatives are usually waiting for them. They should not be inconvenienced any more than is necessary.

The first question you should ask yourself when you are required to sign a death certificate is 'Can I write it?' Usually you are managing the patient and the diagnosis is clear; if the death is expected then the underlying condition is usually known and the cause of death is obvious. If you do not know the cause of death, or cannot make a reasonable assumption, you should discuss this with your seniors and a post-mortem examination should be made. This is done through the coroner, who will request the post-mortem on your behalf. This must always be discussed with deceased patients' relatives, which can be difficult, so proceed with compassion but always explain the importance and that a certificate cannot be issued without a cause of death.

There are other reasons why a death should be referred to the coroner. The Office of National Statistics has given a list of these situations.

When writing a death certificate, do not use abbreviations. Write dates in words and write legibly – use capitals. The cause of death is split into several sections:

- Ia – Disease or condition directly leading to death: this is the direct cause of death, e.g. myocardial infarction, bronchopneumonia. The 'failures', e.g. acute renal failure, hepatic failure or congestive cardiac failure can be used but must be qualified in section Ib with an underlying diagnosis.
- Ib – Other disease or condition, if any leading to Ia: this is the underlying disease condition, e.g. chronic obstructive airways disease, ischaemic heart disease.
- Ic – Other disease or condition, if any, leading to Ib: if any underlying condition encompasses all of the other categories, then this should be included here. This might include conditions that could be in sections Ia and Ib, for example:
  - Ia bronchopneumonia
    Ib chronic obstructive airways disease
  - Ia septicaemia
    Ib bronchopneumonia
    Ic acute myeloid leukaemia.
- II – Other significant conditions contributing to death but not related to the disease or condition causing it: this is any other significant comorbidity, for example:
  - Ia respiratory failure
    Ib disseminated carcinomatosis
    Ic carcinoma of prostate
  - II chronic obstructive airways disease.

Avoid diagnoses such as 'old age' – the patient might have been old but was in hospital for a reason. Do not make up a diagnosis if you are not sure – contact your seniors or discuss it with a pathologist or the coroner if you are in any doubt.

Cremation forms

As with death certificates, the expeditious completion of cremation forms is essential to allow cremation to take place without added delay and distress to the family of the deceased. It is often a good idea to fill in your part of the cremation form at the same time as the death certificate, and with the prevalence of shift systems within medicine nowadays, this is doubly important. Your successor might not have looked after the patient and will therefore be unable to fill in the cremation form.

The following are a few points worth noting when filling in cremation forms:

- You must fill in all the boxes for your part (first part) of the cremation form. Make sure that the causes of death that you put down are exactly the same as those on the death certificate.

- You must see the body after death. Go and visit the morgue, check the face and name tag, and feel for a pacemaker on the chest wall. Check in the notes that no radioactive implants have been used.

- You are asked for the mode of death. This is a somewhat artificial construct, but if death was sudden, use 'syncope', if comatose, use 'coma' and if death was a slow decline struggling against illness, use 'exhaustion'.

- Check the notes carefully to ensure that no operation was conducted within a year of death. If it was, speak to your seniors.

You will receive a fee for each cremation form that you fill in. This fee is due to you, although you can waive it if you wish – you will need to discuss this with the funeral directors. Some hospitals take part of the fee as a spurious 'administrative expense'; still other hospitals funnel cremation fees into the doctors' mess. If you receive the money, keep a note of it – the Inland Revenue need to know about your cremation fees and will chase you if you don't declare them.

What to say

Consenting patients

In an ideal world, as a foundation doctor you would not obtain consent for operations and procedures; this task is most appropriately done by the person who will be carrying out the procedure. However, you will still be called upon to explain procedures and obtain consent, and the medicolegal aspects of obtaining valid informed consent become ever more stringent as the years pass. Check your local guidance, as well as the GMC guidance on obtaining informed consent.

Do you know what the procedure is? Go and see the operations and procedures that you will be consenting people for. If you don't know what the procedure involves, you should not consent the patient.

Do you know what the complications are? Nowadays, it is a good idea to know what the complication rates within your unit are. In a couple of years' time, you will need to know the complication rates for the operator who will perform the procedure.

How should you explain the procedure? You will find that you develop a 'patter' for the more common procedures. Do not let this hinder your ability to communicate effectively – everyone needs a slightly different way of explaining things:

- avoid jargon
- start with why the procedure is needed
- explain the type of anaesthetic (if known; otherwise leave this to the anaesthetist)
- explain the procedure
- explain what will happen after the procedure; tell patients where they will be and whether they will have tubes sticking out of them
- explain how long it will take to recover
- explain the complications

It is very helpful to use pictures to explain procedures. Draw a picture on the back of the consent form (to prove that you have used pictures) or give patients a drawing.

How much should you tell patients? It used to be taught that anything below a 1% risk of serious injury or death did not need to be disclosed to patients, in case they were frightened unnecessarily from having vital procedures. Ethics and expectations have changed and the medicolegal climate is now moving towards an expectation that patients are told any fact that might conceivably affect their decision to consent. Thus, all risks of death or serious injury should probably be disclosed. Be guided by the patients – if they want to know, tell them.

You don't think your patient is competent to consent Do not force patients to sign the form if you are not sure that they are competent. Some problems are easily solved – make sure that any hearing aid is switched on and that the patient's reading glasses are to hand.

Confused patients or those who are too ill to give consent are a different matter. The law states that such patients (if adults) can be treated under common law without informed consent provided that such treatment is in the patient's best interests. No-one other than the patient can give consent to treatment.

Most hospitals have forms that relatives or other doctors can sign in such circumstances. Relatives cannot give consent on behalf of adults (parents can on behalf of children, however) and such forms have no legal standing. Seeking assent from relatives is, however, good ethical practice but the needs of the adult patient should always prevail over the wishes of relatives. The exception is a patient with a relative who holds welfare power of attorney.

Referring patients

There is nothing more irritating than receiving a referral from someone who doesn't tell a coherent story. You will undoubtedly have to refer many patients for opinions from other doctors; the following are some pointers as to how to get it right.

REFERRING BY TELEPHONE

- Make sure that you know the patient's history well, the reason for referral and what outcome you expect from the referral. Ask your seniors if you are unsure. Have the notes in front of you when you call.

- Refer in good time. Don't leave referrals to the end of the day, especially on Friday afternoon, unless it is unavoidable.

- Introduce yourself on the telephone and check that you are speaking to the right person. Even better, see if you can find them in person.

- Ask for their help. Briefly explain the main features of the case and state why you are phoning them. Do not ramble through a full history and examination.

- Record your conversation in the notes and leave a short précis of the case in the notes, along with the latest investigation results.

REFERRING BY LETTER

Occasionally, you might have to dictate or write a referral letter. The same principles apply; give a brief account of the history, examination, investigations and course to date, and frame a question to be answered, e.g. 'Would this woman benefit from surgery?' Look at some referral letters to get an idea of how it is done and practise using a dictaphone (perhaps to do the occasional discharge summary – your registrar will probably thank you profusely).

Breaking bad news

There is no easy way to break bad news and there is no single right way of doing it. Breaking bad news is – by its very nature – a painful process, both for the recipient and the giver of the news. There is no shame at all in showing emotion during the process – indeed, the day you stop feeling anything when you break bad news is the day you should leave medicine.

There are a few ways that you can make the task of breaking bad news less traumatic for the recipient:

- Find out how much the patient knows or suspects. This is easier if you have got to know the patient or relatives beforehand.

- Select a time and place where you have privacy and time – do not give bad news in the middle of the ward round. Consider a private room rather than just pulling the curtains round, and give your bleep to someone.

- Ask a member of the nursing staff to accompany you and – if the patient wishes – a close relative.

- Ensure that you know the plan and the prognosis before you start.

- Try and break the bad news in stages. Ideally, the stage should have been set in the days leading up to the breaking of the news.

- Avoid jargon. If the patient has cancer, say 'cancer' – not tumour, malignancy, growth or any other euphemism.

- Be frank but not overly precise. You don't actually know how long the patient will survive.

- Always leave the person with some hope, but ensure that this is not delivered frivolously. 'Cheer up, it might never happen' is clearly not going to help matters.

- No matter how busy you are, give enough time to the person. Don't keep sneaking a look at your watch.

- Don't be afraid of offering physical contact, but don't feel that you have to offer this.

- Crying, shouting, anger and laughter are all emotional responses that can be precipitated by bad news – as is silence. Give time for the recipient to express any emotions and don't feel that every silence has to be filled with your meaningless babble.

- Deliver information a bit at a time. People in shock do not remember much (another reason to have nursing staff and relatives present). The recipient will not be able to remember the details of the side-effects of chemotherapy if you explain them at the same time as delivering the diagnosis of cancer.

- Finish by letting the recipient know that you will be around to answer any questions or to talk further. Written information can also be very helpful.

It is a good idea to go back later and check how much of the information the recipient took in. Better still, do this before the oncologists or surgeons come to talk about further therapy.

Talking to relatives

Good communication extends well beyond talking to your patients – keeping the relatives in the picture is not only courteous but helps to facilitate discharge and improves the care and support that your patients will receive both in and out of hospital. The following are a few points to bear in mind:

- Always ask patients whether they mind you speaking to their relatives.

- Involve the relatives early, and keep them involved. Be proactive; don't wait for them to come and find you.

- Listen to the concerns of relatives, for instance, about the ability of older, frail patients to manage on their own.

- Don't forget that relatives are carers and that they often need support to keep caring for your patient.

- In large families, agree on one person to act as the conduit for discussion. This can reduce the amount of time that you spend repeating yourself.

- Don't forget that families have their own internal dynamics. Two halves of a family might not speak to each other and some relatives might not want what your patient wants. Despite this, don't be cynical about people's motives – not all family squabbles are about father's last will and testament. If things start to get complicated, get your seniors involved.

- Relatives can get angry about perceived delays in diagnosis, treatment, discharge, or about the fact that their relative is dying. Grief, fear and guilt can all play a part and the best policy is to listen a lot, stick to the facts and write everything down. If genuine mistakes have been made, apologize, but do not feel that you should make promises that you cannot personally keep, e.g. dates of discharge, times of investigations.

- Tell your patients how much their relatives know, and vice versa. This eases communication within the family.
- Some families wish to withhold bad news from the patient and will ask you not to tell the patient the diagnosis or prognosis. You are not bound by their wishes, but seek to persuade the family that disclosure would be the best policy, rather than barging in and breaking the news without the family onside.
- Write a summary of your conversations with relatives in the notes.

Managing your work

Time management

Being a foundation doctor can seem rather like being a hamster on a wheel; the harder you work, the more there is to do. The more patients you discharge, the more come in to your ward for clerking. Every time you get close to completing a task, someone bleeps you away.

This state of affairs, if uncontrolled, can lead to tremendous inefficiency (nothing is completed) and great personal dissatisfaction, either as a result of feeling that the job isn't done properly or because of having to work later and later. The solution is time management: remember, tasks can be divided into the four types shown in Fig. 13.

Clearly urgent, important tasks must be attended to immediately. What often stops effective use of time however, is spending too much of your time doing seemingly urgent but somewhat less important tasks. Such tasks have to be done but care should be taken to avoid interrupting other activities every time a new task crops up. In short – prioritize.

One of the keys to job satisfaction, not to mention personal growth and providing the best service possible to your patients, is spending enough time on important but non-urgent tasks. It is not a luxury to go and read about medical advances, a new disease or drug, or find out about something that your patient has asked you about. All these are part of your job, and you need to ensure that you spend time on these important but less urgent activities. If that means delaying some urgent, less important business once in a while, so be it.

Teamwork Scratch your colleagues' backs and they will (usually) scratch yours. Whether this means taking some forms down to X-ray when they go, or holding a bleep when they go to the library, give and take within your team and with your foundation colleagues can make life a lot easier.

Ward rounds - preparing, going on them, running them

Think for a moment what the purpose of a ward round is – it is an opportunity to go over histories and examinations, to review the latest test results and – most importantly – it is the time when many decisions are taken about management. It should also, of course, be a time for communicating with your patients. So what does your consultant need to make those decisions on the ward round?

Four jobs commonly performed by a foundation doctor		
	Urgent	Non-urgent
Important	Patient fitting	Reading up about a rare disease you have encountered
Less important	Filling in discharge summary	Rewriting drug chart

Fig. 13 The four types of job commonly performed by a foundation year 1 doctor (F1).

- Ready access to the history and the examination is important, so make sure that the notes are all ready for inspection and that you know at least an outline of everyone's story.
- Ideally, the patient needs to be present – this is not always easy, but if possible liaise with the nursing staff and with investigations to ensure that patients are available to be seen. Know where on the wards the patients are – this saves a tremendous amount of time. A list for each member of the team is useful.
- The consultant will certainly need access to the latest investigations – the bloods, X-rays and special tests, especially those discussed on the last ward round. It is your job – no-one else's – to ensure that these results are immediately to hand. Write them in the notes – a lot easier than fiddling with the computer. Use a cumulative results chart, especially with conditions such as renal failure or chronic sepsis.

It is a good idea to at least try and steer the ward round. You are in charge – kick off the discussion about each patient, recount a very brief précis of the history and progress, and introduce the latest results. Give your team verbal prompts to help them remember who the patient is and remind your consultant as to what decisions need to be made, e.g. next investigations, starting new medication, when to discharge. It is also your job to write in the notes – don't assume someone else will do this and don't attempt to wait until after the round to write in the notes. As the round progresses, make a list of jobs on your patient list. If any member of your team appears to be underutilized, give them something to do – writing TTOs, X-ray cards or adding drugs to prescription charts. A ward round is a team enterprise.

Once the round is over, go through your list of jobs. Prioritize – get the urgent tests done first, then TTOs then routine jobs.

Discharges/TTOs (to-take-out medicines)

Nothing causes more grief among patients, relatives and nursing staff than delays in discharge because discharge medications are not ready. Although you cannot speed up the pharmacy dispensary, you can help the process by writing TTOs at the earliest opportunity – think about what you would want to happen if you were a patient who had been told that you could go home that afternoon. If possible, find out who is likely to go home the day before the ward round and write the TTOs then. Some patients will have medications changed on the ward round; write their TTOs on the round (or get your colleagues to do so). Not every patient needs TTOs – check to see if the patient has enough medicines at home.

Ensure that at least brief discharge details accompany the patient home – usually on a copy of the TTO. A dictated discharge summary usually follows later; your registrar is usually responsible for producing this.

Ordering tests

You will spend a lot of your time as a foundation doctor ordering tests, often at someone else's request. The first thing to ensure, therefore, is that you know why the test is being ordered:

- what is the differential diagnosis?
- what are the clinical features?
- why this test and not some other test?
- why now and not later (for urgent tests)?
- most important of all, how will the results change your management?

If you don't know why you are ordering a test – ask someone. You cannot give a rationale for wanting a test if you don't know why it is being requested, and when it comes to talking to radiologists, endoscopists and other specialists, it is essential that you know why you are asking for something. When ordering a test:

- Don't just put a vague explanation such as 'collapse' on your request forms. The more information you can give the labs or radiology, the more useful information will come back to you.

- Order tests early. Find out when the phlebotomy rounds are, get the forms in well before this, and try and anticipate what your team will order next – this saves having to request add-on tests (labs hate these) or taking more blood. Similarly, get your ultrasound, CT and X-ray requests in before lunchtime; this will probably save you a day at least and, if a slot comes up in the afternoon, your patient could be first in the queue.

- Finally, go and talk to people face to face. Get to know the radiologists, echo technicians and ultrasonographers. Ask their opinion. Make them feel valued and use their skills. They are not just skivvies employed to do your bidding. Face-to-face contact will often open doors and speed things up in ways that are impossible with an impersonal telephone call.

Being on call

Eat It is very easy to forget to eat when you are on call but, if you are hungry, your performance – in terms of speed, judgement and manual dexterity – will suffer. You will also feel tetchy and hard-done-by; not qualities likely to impress your patients or your colleagues! There is very rarely anything so urgent that it cannot wait for 10 min while you eat a sandwich or a microwave meal.

Drink Similarly, it is easy to forget to drink and, if you are on call for 12 hours, you will lose quite a lot of fluid. Hospitals are often hot and you are usually rushing around. Dehydrated doctors are not effective doctors; make sure a bottle of water is on hand.

Sleep If you have the chance to get to bed, do so – unless it is likely to be for less than an hour (some people feel worse after half an hour's sleep). Don't sit there watching TV; you don't know when you will be called in the middle of the night, so use the time to sleep when you can. Short naps at night can improve concentration.

Comfort Don't forget to visit the toilet – this might sound stupid but it will happen, and you cannot concentrate when you are desperate to urinate.

See your ward patients early in the day if you are still scheduled to cover a ward. If you are scheduled to do clinics on your on-call day, insist that they are cancelled. You cannot do both jobs at once and it is unfair on your clinic patients if you are unable to give them 100% of your attention.

Hospital at night Many hospitals are now running Hospital at Night teams to cover late evening and overnight. This is a rather different way of working than you will be used to during the day, as you will be working alongside senior medical staff (usually a registrar) but also a senior nurse, who will usually assess calls and allocate jobs to you. A few pointers to making Hospital at Night work are:

- Make sure you attend handover and have a full list of potentially unwell patients and jobs that need to be done.

- Try and meet up with the rest of the team at least once and preferably twice during the night.

- Ask for help. You will often be covering patients that you don't know in specialities that you have little experience of. You have senior staff on your team; use them.

- Remember that the nursing staff on the team are much more experienced than you; respect their opinion and if they ask for you to attend a patient urgently, do it!

- Make sure that you attend handover in the morning, and hand over everyone that you have been involved in, no matter how small the problem was. Similarly, if unwell people did not give concern overnight, hand this over too.

MANAGING SHIFT WORK AT NIGHT

Shift working at nights is arduous, but there are a number of things that you can do to help yourself cope:

- Get plenty of sleep before you start a run of nights.

- Bright lights at work will make you feel more awake.

- Make sure you eat three meals a day.

- Don't drive if you are too tired in the morning.

- Wear sunglasses on the way home to avoid bright light tricking your brain into thinking it is time to be awake.

- Go to bed as soon as you get home, in a dark room. Do not stay up watching daytime TV.

Bleep management

The bleep, exciting as it might seem when you are a medical student, is the most tyrannical device ever invented from the point of view of doctors. Put it in its place as a tool, not as your master:

- Ensure that each ward that you cover has a board where non-urgent tasks can be written. Make sure that you check the board regularly. If you are still bleeped a lot about seemingly non-urgent tasks, discuss the matter with the staff concerned – work together to solve their problem and you will be bleeped less.

- Answer your bleep as promptly as you can but don't allow it to interfere with important tasks such as talking to patients or relatives. If you have an important conversation that you need to conduct, especially one involving bad news, leave your bleep elsewhere – with the ward clerk or with a colleague.

- Do not be tempted to answer your bleep when you have left the hospital – this is your free time. If you are tempted, take the battery out of the bleep when you leave the hospital.

- Your education time should be bleep-free. Give your bleep to someone else, e.g. the postgraduate office.

Remember – the bleep is a tool. If it constantly interrupts your other tasks, your education and your free time, you will not work well, learn well or live well – and you will thus be a less good doctor.

Teamwork

Almost all work in the world is performed in teams, and medicine is no exception. So why do doctors still work so dysfunctionally in a team environment? A few tips for successful teamwork are as follows:

- Acknowledge the skills and experience of others in the team, especially nursing and allied health professionals. They know more than you, and have been in practice longer than you.

- Treat others as you would want them to treat you. Respect is a two-way street.
- Give credit and praise to the team when things go well.
- Acknowledge your errors, and never try to blame others. If something goes wrong, the team takes responsibility.
- Make time to get to know your fellow team members. They are human beings too.
- Talk to each other. Lack of communication is the single biggest cause of team dysfunction.
- Ask for advice, and ask how you can do things better.
- Don't forget that you are all working toward the same goal – the good of your patient. It is not about turf wars, demarcation or empire building.

Education

Your foundation posts are training posts – the GMC looks upon foundation training very much as an extension of medical school. Education is your right and you should not let service commitments stand in the way of receiving education and training. Although this is clearly easier said than done, there are a few things that you can do to help ensure that you are educated:

- Don't take your bleep into lectures and educational seminars. Not only is it rude to those presenting but, if you are contactable, someone will try and contact you – no matter how many times you ask them not to. Give your bleep to another member of your team, or to the postgraduate office.
- Plan your working day so that your routine jobs are done by the time the education session takes place.
- Keep a list of conditions seen and managed, procedures done, dilemmas faced. Start from day 1 in the job.
- Meet your educational supervisor and explain what you want. This – of course – necessitates thinking about your career goals and what you want to gain from each foundation post. Push to meet your supervisor early in the job; certainly within the first 3 weeks – time flies!
- Get to the library; little and often is usually the best plan. Even if it is only reading the *BMJ* once a week, try and keep reading – perhaps read up on an interesting case you have seen, or find the evidence behind a course of action that your team has taken.
- Get auditing. Although audit can be tedious, it can give you insight into many aspects of the process of care – why we do what we do – and a good audit can help to effect real change in patient care. Start early and don't rely on the audit department of your hospital; it is usually grossly overstretched and far too slow to allow you to finish an audit within 6 months.
- Offer to present. Do this whether or not you are a natural public speaker; it is good practice and a necessary skill to acquire anywhere in the working world. Also, find out if you can get help with other skills such as interview skills, computing skills, etc. If your hospital doesn't run courses in these subjects for foundation doctors ask why not.

Maintaining life balance

The change to a working culture, long hours and stressful situations all play a part in turning the average foundation doctor into a walking zombie. Many foundation doctors work excessive hours, sleep badly, drink to excess and talk about medicine to the exclusion of everything else – we know from personal experience. This is clearly unhealthy and if such a way of life continues for several years, job dissatisfaction, poor health and ruined relationships become likely.

Keep a sense of balance in your life. You work long hours in a hospital – so get out of it when you can, especially at weekends. Try and eat healthily, and drink in moderation; not only will you feel healthier, you will work more efficiently. Get some exercise – run, swim, or just walk.

Remember that there is more to life than work. Try and ensure that you don't just socialize with other medical staff; this might allow you to let off steam but it also leads to a one-dimensional intellectual existence and tends to lead to a self-perpetuating negative view of the world as seen through medical eyes and medical eyes only. Keep up at least one of your former hobbies, keep in regular touch with your family and keep a supply of good music on hand!

Preparing patients for theatre

Preoperative assessments

Most preoperative clerkings take place in a preadmission clinic a week or so before the operation. The purpose of these is to assess the patient regarding fitness for theatre, perform baseline screening tests, obtain written consent and answer any last-minute questions the patient might have. The last of these points can only be dealt with satisfactorily if you have a reasonable idea of what the operation entails, as well as an awareness of potential postoperative complications. The clerking should include:

- History: a brief history of the patient's illness including a summary of the symptoms and any relevant test result (including their dates).

- Any significant medical history that might influence the patient's fitness for theatre: e.g. cardiovascular or respiratory problems such as angina or COPD. Significant arthritis, especially in the neck, is also relevant, particularly if the patient requires intubation.

- Any previous anaesthetic problems and a full allergy and drug history.

- Examination: a brief but thorough examination of the cardiovascular, respiratory and abdominal systems should be made. This should include vital signs including blood pressure. Any relevant other examination should also be made, e.g. peripheral pulses for vascular patients.

- Investigations: all patients require FBC and U+Es preoperatively. LFTs and clotting screen (INR) should be done on:
  - any patient with history of liver dysfunction or alcohol excess
  - any patient where there is a suspected malignancy, e.g. colectomy, thyroid resection
  - any patient undergoing biliary surgery.

- Amylase should be performed pre- and postoperatively in any patient undergoing biliary or pancreatic surgery (including ERCP).

- Blood products: minor surgery such as routine hernia repairs and varicose veins do not require any blood products to be requested; most other surgery should have a group and save sample sent at preadmission clinic. It is also important to send another sample on the day the patient is admitted for surgery because the blood bank will not keep the original sample more than 2–3 days; it is used to screen for antibodies but the second sample is needed to cross-match any blood products required.

There are usually local guidelines for cross-matching blood for surgery, but here are some guides:

- Most bowel/vascular/endocrine surgery: cross-match 2 units.
- Major surgery, e.g. bowel resection: cross-match 4 units.
- Major vascular surgery, e.g. AAA repair: cross-match 4 units.
- Chest X-ray: should be performed on:
  - patients with any history of lung disease
  - patients where metastatic spread needs to be excluded
  - patients over the age of 55.
- Routine chest X-rays are unnecessary in patients under 55 if they are well.

- There is virtually no indication for preoperative chest X-rays in children.
- The chest X-ray should be looked at prior to the patient coming into theatre – it is very embarrassing to miss something and to be contacted by the anaesthetist afterwards!
- ECGs: should be performed in patients over the age of 65 and in all patients who have a cardiac history, diabetes or hypertension.

Drug charts

As well as their normal drugs, patients undergoing surgery require additional drugs:

- Pre-meds: these are usually taken care of by the anaesthetist but some surgery might require drugs, e.g. antibiotics, vitamin K prior to surgery. You should familiarize yourself with local policy.
- DVT prophylaxis: TED stockings and low molecular weight heparin, e.g. enoxaparin, are fairly standard for most surgery to prevent DVT and PE. These need to be prescribed. Give heparin at 6 p.m. This allows an epidural to be given safely for major abdominal procedures. The first dose can be given at induction in some procedures.
- Antiemetics: cyclizine 50 mg IV, IM or orally is a good antiemetic and can be prescribed on an as-needed basis.
- Analgesia: there is no need for a patient ever to be in pain postoperatively so adequate analgesia is vital. For most major surgery, the anaesthetist will prescribe a PCA pump (patient-controlled analgesia) and will manage it in the postoperative period. Make sure that antiemetics and analgesia (e.g. morphine) are prescribed for when the pump is discontinued. Simple analgesia should be prescribed according to the analgesic ladder with the addition of NSAIDs (where not contraindicated by allergy, peptic ulcer disease, heart failure or renal impairment) for musculoskeletal pain.

Written consent

As stated previously, the reason for seeing the patient early is to consent them for surgery. It is important that you are aware of the procedures involved, common and important complications and the usual length of stay in hospital. If you are unaware of these facts, ask your seniors. It is very difficult to talk to a patient in ignorance and it is not fair on the patient; also, consent will be invalid because it is not informed consent. Remember also to briefly mention anaesthetic complications, although most patients will be seen by an anaesthetist preoperatively.

Diabetic patients

Patients with diabetes pose specific problems when they go to theatre. They are slightly more prone to infection and their wound healing can be slower than normal. They also tend to come with a multitude of additional medical problems, e.g. ischaemic heart disease and renal problems. The main problem tends to be good blood sugar management perioperatively and postoperatively.

Patients on tablets or diet control can be reasonably put nil by mouth from midnight the night before their surgery. Their morning tablets should be omitted and a close eye kept on their BMs (1–2-hourly). The normal IV infusion of normal saline should be started, although IV dextrose can be used in the event of hypoglycaemia.

An insulin sliding scale	
BM	Insulin (U/h)
> 17	6
11 –17	4
7 –11	2
4 –7	1
< 4	0.5

Fig. 14 An example of a sliding insulin scale. 50 U Actrapid in 50 mL normal saline.

Patients on insulin should be managed slightly differently. They should take their normal insulin the night before surgery and check their BMs regularly in the morning. In hospital they should be started on an IV infusion of dextrose and an IV insulin sliding scale (see below) – an alternative is the GKI (glucose, potassium and insulin) regime, where all three are given in a single bag. There is no place for subcutaneous insulin sliding scales. BMs should be measured every hour and supplemental dextrose used if the patient becomes hypoglycaemic. A suggested sliding scale is shown in Fig. 14.

Patients on warfarin

Patients on warfarin also pose a problem for surgery. The crucial question is 'why is the patient on warfarin?'.

Patients on warfarin for prosthetic heart valves should never have their warfarin stopped without heparin cover. They should ideally be admitted a day or so before surgery, their warfarin stopped and IV heparin started to provide ongoing anticoagulation. This can then be stopped during surgery and restarted afterwards. If you are in doubt, discuss such patients with your seniors and your local cardiologist or haematologist.

Patients on warfarin for thromboembolic disease or atrial fibrillation (AF) should be discussed with a member of the medical team on an individual basis so that their risk can be ascertained. Generally, patients in AF can have warfarin stopped for the perioperative period and restarted later.

All patients who have had their warfarin stopped should have an urgent INR sent preoperatively, with the result available before the patient goes to theatre.

Nil by mouth (NBM)

NBM means no food from midnight prior to the operation. It does not mean that patients cannot take their normal medication. This is particularly important for cardiac drugs. Patients are allowed to have up to 60 mL of fluid for tablet taking. The obvious exception to this is diabetic patients on oral hypoglycaemic agents who are nil by mouth – the tablets can be omitted in the absence of food.

IV fluids

Preoperative All patients should have an IV infusion of normal saline before going to theatre. This is to prevent dehydration before surgery. Normal saline is the fluid of choice (although dextrose can be used, particularly in diabetics) running in 4–6-hourly bags. Try to avoid potassium supplementation because this bag might need to be run in very quickly if the patient becomes hypotensive during anaesthetic induction.

Postoperative Postoperatively, the vast majority of surgical patients will need lots of fluids. Surgery, particularly bowel surgery, causes massive fluid loss into the gut, and this needs to be replaced. A guide is the amount of fluid given peri-operatively. Look at the anaesthetic chart; for example if 6 L of fluid was given during the operation, the patient will probably need two 4-hourly bags of normal saline followed by a litre over 6 h and then a litre over 8 h. Again, normal saline is the fluid of choice, especially to replace losses. Normal saline can be alternated with 5% dextrose for maintenance fluids – remember to add in extra normal saline to replace losses from vomiting, diarrhoea and wound drains. U+Es should be measured regularly and potassium supplements given as appropriate.

Postoperative complications

Complications for specific surgery will not be dealt with here; you should discuss these with your seniors. There are, however, some common postoperative problems that can occur in any patient. Exclude these common causes and document them.

FEVER

The crucial question is 'is the patient unwell?' If a patient is well (ask yourself 'does this patient look well?' 'does this patient have good oxygenation, pulse < 100, respiratory rate < 20, urine output > 30 mL/h?') then only examination and cultures are needed. Treatment with antibiotics should only be for a known infection or in a sick patient with best-guess antibiotics. Common sites for infection postoperatively are:

- Chest: examine the patient's chest, check vital signs and O_2 saturations, and perform arterial blood gases if necessary. Perform a chest X-ray.
- Urinary tract: check urine dipstick for blood/protein, and examine the patient particularly for loin tenderness. UTIs are common after removal of urinary catheter.
- Wounds: check wound and drain sites for cellulitis and collections.
- Check WCC and CRP, as well as blood cultures and relevant specimens for culture, before commencing any antibiotics.
- DVT/PE: thromboembolic complications can give a mild fever. Examine the patient's calves for swelling and tenderness, and examine the respiratory system for any signs of a PE. Perform a chest X-ray and arterial blood gases breathing air if there is any doubt.
- Blood transfusion: mild pyrexias can be seen during and after blood transfusions. These should be observed, the blood slowed down and paracetamol given if appropriate.

BREATHLESSNESS

- Give O_2 and analgesia while you investigate the cause.
- PE and pneumonia should be excluded. Examine the patient, check O_2 saturations, blood gases on air as well as an ECG.

- If the patient has had a central line inserted either by internal jugular or subclavian approach, then consider pneumothorax in your differential diagnosis.
- If a PE is clinically suspected, give treatment with IV heparin – this should be discussed with your senior, and preferably with the medical team, because treating postoperative patients with heparin might cause significant bleeding.
- Wheeze might be due to bronchoconstriction or pulmonary oedema. Get a chest X-ray and try nebulized salbutamol while you wait for this.

CHEST PAIN

- Give O_2 and analgesia.
- PE and MI/acute coronary syndrome should be excluded. Examine the patient, check O_2 saturations and blood gases on air. Do an ECG.
- Look for any signs of ongoing ischaemia or MI – call for senior help if these are present.
- Patients with known coronary disease can develop angina as a result of anaemia as a result of poor oxygenation due to the low haemoglobin. This should be treated with O_2 and transfusion. Troponin or CK will not be of use during the episode; do a troponin 6–12 h later. CK is often raised from the surgery itself.

TACHYCARDIA

The most common reasons will be moderate hypovolaemia and inadequate analgesia. Make sure the patient is comfortable and give fluids. Your task is then to exclude serious causes. Check the patient's blood pressure and perform an ECG. If the patient is tachycardic and hypotensive, the most likely cause is bleeding and you should call for senior help while resuscitating the patient with IV colloid. Other causes of shock should be considered (e.g. sepsis, massive PE) but the initial management is no different.

If the patient has a normal blood pressure and has a sinus tachycardia, consider:

- infection
- PE
- bleeding
- inadequate analgesia
- dehydration

Patients commonly go into uncontrolled atrial fibrillation postoperatively. This can be due to dehydration, electrolyte imbalance or the presence of infection or pulmonary embolus. All of these should be excluded (FBC, U+Es, blood gases on air and ECG) and, if necessary, the patient should be rate-controlled with digoxin – 500 µg over 30 min IV is a good place to start, followed by 250 µg IV 6–12 h later. Refer a patient who remains in AF to the medical team for investigation and further management.

POOR URINE OUTPUT

This is usually due to dehydration. Most patients require large amounts of fluid post-operatively and if they become dry, their urine output decreases. Thus the treatment is rehydration. U+Es should be checked. Other causes, such as a blocked catheter, should also be excluded – feel for a bladder and flush the catheter. If initial rehydration (e.g. 500 mL colloid followed by 1 L normal saline over 1 h) is ineffective, discuss with your senior.

If the patient has poor urine output and pulmonary oedema, call for senior help immediately.

What to do when things go wrong

When things go wrong in your life

There is a reasonable chance that a major life event will happen during your foundation years. This might be a bereavement, the break-up of a close relationship or the diagnosis of a serious illness. There is a great temptation to struggle on at work despite the extra pressure 'because you're a doctor and that's what doctors do'. True – that's what doctors often do, and that is one reason why they have much higher suicide, divorce and alcoholism rates than most other professionals. When something goes badly wrong outside your working life, it is time to look after number one first. Sounds too difficult? Then think that you are failing to give your patients the best and safest service that you can if you are burdened with illness, or are preoccupied with grief.

Talk to your friends. Tell your consultant. If your consultant is unsympathetic, tell your educational supervisor or head of department. Tell them as early as you can, so that they have time to make arrangements to cover your leave. You are not letting your colleagues down by taking time off in these circumstances; on the contrary, they will appreciate being told and the sooner you can return to peak performance, the happier they will all be.

Work stress

Life is full of chronic stress, which is the condition that results when stressors cannot be controlled or resolved. Life as a foundation doctor is even more full of stress than normal, and it can often be difficult as one of the most junior members of staff to exercise much in the way of control over these stressors.

Some foundation doctors try and combat stress by working ever harder and longer; others turn to the bottle. Neither is a satisfactory solution and both are likely to make the problem worse, not better. So what can you do?

- Make sure that you have enough relaxation time and activities outside of the work environment.
- Take physical exercise and leave enough time for a good night's sleep.
- Try and identify the sources of stress and work with others to alleviate them. Don't get on well with the ward sister? Try having a discussion about how you can change or how you can be more helpful. No time for lunch? Cooperate with your colleagues to hold each other's bleeps.

Bullying

Although the culture of bullying used to be an integral part of medicine, the situation is slowly changing. Nevertheless, bullying is still rife in some areas of medicine. It is always unacceptable. Every trust should have a policy regarding bullying and harrassment – if you are being bullied, look at the policy and talk to someone. Once again, your educational supervisor might be a good person. Is there a pastoral tutor in the hospital who you could talk to?

Many junior doctors do not talk about bullying for fear that they will not get a reference. Ask yourself what a reference from a bully says about your capacity and willingness to get a job. Are you really that desperate? If you are good enough, you don't need that reference. There is always someone else who can give you a reference, and if your next set of employers aren't very understanding of this, are they the sort of people that you want to be working for anyway? Bear in mind that the wide range of jobs that you do as a foundation doctor means that a problem with a single supervisor can be countered by references and evidence of competency from all your other supervisors.

Whistleblowing

The GMC is quite clear that if you discover that a colleague is acting in a way that is detrimental to the interests of patients, you have a duty to report such behaviour. It is no longer the case that 'you don't grass on your colleagues'; such behaviour is not for the profession of medicine.

Before speaking out, however, be very sure that you have solid evidence with which to back up your case. Even better, talk to your colleagues and see if they are aware of the problem. Note down times, dates, specifics of incidents – but beware that you do not engage in any behaviour that might be construed as libellous, slanderous, criminal, or that breaches patient confidentiality.

Who to talk to? – a difficult question. If the problem lies outside your department, talk to your consultant or to the medical director of your unit. Problems within your unit are politically and personally more difficult; if possible, try and find a senior confidante outside your unit, perhaps the postgraduate tutor for your hospital. Sometimes, you might find that the problem is institution-wide; if so, your defence organization might be the best people to talk to. You can always talk to the GMC directly if you find other avenues are blocked.

Once you have brought problems to the attention of people in senior places, do not feel that you need to sort out the whole problem by yourself – you are not expected to have to do this as a very junior doctor. Whistleblowing is very stressful and can make going to work an unpleasant experience. Nevertheless, you have a professional and moral obligation to whistleblow if needed, and it does not automatically mean the end of your reference, your career or your happiness. Your actions could potentially benefit hundreds of patients.

Adverse incidents

Healthcare is immensely complex and, as with any system involving human beings, things will go wrong. An adverse incident is any event that causes the performance of the healthcare system to deviate from optimum. You will find that this happens hundreds of times a week – from an X-ray getting lost to a patient suffering anaphylaxis from a known drug allergy. Most adverse incidents cause little or no long-term harm; a few result in the death of a patient.

Every adverse incident is a chance to change practice and improve our healthcare system. Sadly, most adverse incidents are either ignored (if no serious harm occurs) or used as a tool to blame an individual. This is not only unfair – most incidents are the result of many factors (e.g. resources, physical layout, training, teamwork) but it also discourages people from reporting and using adverse incidents to improve practice.

So what should you do if something goes wrong? First of all, don't ignore it – even if it is a small problem such as X-rays always getting lost. One day, a lost X-ray will end-up influencing a course of management that could result in a patient's death. Second, report it. The recently formed National Patient Safety Agency has rolled out its incident-reporting system to hospitals in England and Wales; drug side-effects should be reported on the yellow cards found at the back of the BNF. Third, go back over the incident and ask yourself how you contributed to it – what you did well, what you would change next time. Could you improve your knowledge? Is there a team-working problem? Did equipment fail? What can you do about these things?

Don't forget that errors and incidents happen to everyone in medicine, so don't feel that you are a failure if something goes wrong. The only failure is if you and your work environment fail to learn from the incident. Conversely, don't judge your colleagues harshly when they experience adverse incidents; it could be your turn tomorrow. Only spectacularly ignorant doctors never commit errors.

Complaints

Like adverse incidents, complaints are frequent and inevitable whenever human beings interact with each other. Some complaints are justified, others less so; just remember that for every unjustified complaint there is another person who didn't complain who probably had excellent grounds to do so. A few simple rules are worth remembering when dealing with complaints:

- Listen. Don't get defensive; just listen and allow the complainant to let off some steam. This is sometimes all that is necessary.
- Try and summarize what the main complaints are, and what the person would like to see done about the complaint.
- Apologize. Don't just sit there and say that it isn't your fault. Apologize on behalf of the organization. Show some empathy.
- Suggest a plan of action – things that you will personally do to try and rectify at least some of the grievances. Stick to the plan, and report back to the complainant. Take some responsibility.

Make sure that you keep extensive and accurate notes of all conversations and other matters relating to the complaint and the healthcare surrounding the complaint.

Do not hesitate to involve senior staff at an early stage; get your consultant involved. Don't try and sort out problems that you have no jurisdiction over, e.g. issues of nursing care. Tell the ward sister or charge nurse about the problem and allow them to address problems in their area of jurisdiction.

Poor communication leads to 90% of complaints, and most complaints can be dealt with at a relatively informal level. Although the existence of any complaint suggests that communication has been suboptimal, further poor communication, defensive attitudes and a failure to take responsibility and be responsve to the wishes of the complainant make things much worse.

The coroner

The coroner (or in Scotland, the Procurator Fiscal) is there to investigate deaths of unknown cause. If in doubt about a death, talk to your consultant and to the coroner's officer; it is much better to err on the side of doubt than to be pulled up by the coroner later on. Most deaths referred to the coroner's officer result in either a death certificate being issued or a coroner's post-mortem followed by a death certificate; inquests are rare.

From time to time patients will die in untoward circumstances and an inquest will be held to ascertain the cause and circumstances of death. An inquest is not about establishing guilt but it is nevertheless a judicial exercise. If you are called to give evidence to an inquest, remember the following points:

- Good notes help a lot. Because you can't always predict who is going to suffer an untoward death, always keep good notes. Ensure that your writing is clear, every entry is signed and dated, that your name is legible and that the patient's name is on every page.

- Involve your consultant early when things go wrong. If the patient has already died, ensure that you discuss what happened with your consultant at the earliest opportunity. Your consultant cannot support you without knowing what is going on.

- If a post-mortem occurs, go to it if you possibly can. It shows interest and concern as to the cause of death and the gravity of the case, displays a willingness to learn from mistakes and might also make the pathologist better-disposed towards you.

- When called to give evidence, dress smartly and conservatively. Look like the professional you are. Stand up, speak up, then shut up. Do not give opinions; stick to the facts. If you can't verify what you are saying, don't say it.

As a junior doctor, you are not expected to face an inquest without support – your consultant is ultimately responsible for the care of the patient. You are, however, a qualified professional and you should be in a position to take responsibility for your actions, and to justify those actions.

Asking for and getting help

It is always better to ask for help before you get into real trouble; this is true for diagnosing patients, performing procedures, or sorting out your personal life or career. The following are a list of some organizations that can give you advice and help on a range of problems and issues.

The first stop for most of the problems you are likely to encounter should be your consultant. If you do not feel as if you can talk to your consultant about your problem, you could try:

- your educational supervisor (if this person is not also your consultant)

- the consultant with responsibility for junior doctors issues or education (ask the personnel department)

Some hospitals have named pastoral contacts that you can talk to; again, ask the personnel department for details.

Useful organizations

British Medical Association. For advice on pay, rotas and working conditions, to name but a few issues. Tel: 020 7387 4499; www.bma.org.uk (see the website for local offices)

Doctors Support Network. Help for doctors with mental health problems. Tel: 07071 223 372; www.dsn.org.uk

General Medical Council. For advice on fitness to practise, regulatory and ethical issues, medical education and more. See the website for telephone numbers; www.gmc-uk.org

Medical Defence Union. Tel: 020 7202 1500; www.the-mdu.com

Medical Protection Society. For help with medicolegal problems or potential medicolegal problems. Tel: 0845 605 4000; www.mps.org.uk

National Counselling Service for Sick Doctors. Tel: 0870 241 0535; www.ncssd.org.uk

Royal Medical Benevolent Fund. Helps doctors who have fallen on financial hardship. Tel: 020 8540 9194; www.rmbf.org

Sick Doctors Trust. Helps doctors with alcohol or drug dependency. Tel: 01252 345 163; www.sick-doctors-trust.co.uk

Foundation programme

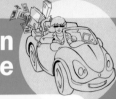

Foundation programme

Introduction

This chapter aims to provide you with information on the new Junior Doctor training programme (the Foundation Programme) from the point of view of someone who has experienced the programme first hand.

Firstly, remember you are still a Junior Doctor. The job you do from day to day is essentially the same as the house officer before you, so, at times, you may feel like an overqualified ECG technician, phlebotomist or secretary. Don't let that upset you. The biggest changes have been in your supervision and your education, and it is important to make the most of these changes in order to learn and progress to the next level.

By the time you read this chapter the first Junior Doctors will have completed years one and two of training. Consequently, the hospitals where you are working will have become adapted to the new system.

Why has the training of doctors changed?

In the past, there were many young doctors who spent years as a senior house officer going from post to post with no end-point or career objective. The primary aim of Modernising Medical Careers (MMC) was to remove the ability to do this and to instead create a greater number of fully trained, highly specialized doctors who can deliver the best care possible. The effect of this change will not be immediate as the first specialist training posts were not appointed until 2007 and those appointed doctors will therefore not complete training for a number of years.

The foundation years are aptly named and their role in MMC is to provide you with a solid foundation from which you can build your future career. Throughout the foundation years your goal is to achieve a number of competencies that will provide you with the basic skills you need to become a competent medical practitioner regardless of the speciality you choose. These skills will range from good communication with patients and colleagues to the competent recognition and management of the acutely unwell patient.

Another aim of the new system is to ensure that training is consistent, no matter which speciality or region you are in. This chapter should reflect on the programme regardless of which Deanery you are working in.

People to know

There are a great number of people involved in running the programme in your Deanery. However, in our experience, there are two particularly important people you need to know:

Foundation tutor

At the start of the first year you will split into groups. What group you are in will depend on the posts you have been allocated. Each tutor looks after a group of Junior Doctors. They oversee your entire training for the 2 years. They are the people who know what you should be doing with regard to your portfolio, and will offer advice about any programme problems you might encounter. They'll also be the ones who will e-mail you towards the end of each post, reminding you about the forms you haven't yet submitted!

Educational supervisor

He or she will change with each post that you do. Generally, they will be the consultant for whom you work in your given post. They are less likely to know about subjects relating to the Foundation Programme but will be able to help you with everyday problems. You can approach them about anything related to that post; for example, clinical dilemmas or any problems with colleagues. They will also value any feedback you can give on ways to improve the programme for the next trainee.

Job selection

The programme gives you the opportunity to experience a variety of specialities that you may otherwise not have had exposure to. You will work through six 4-month posts over the 2 years. You will have some say in the choice of rotation, but it is difficult to accommodate everybody's first choice. The posts that you work in will include a 4-month general medical and a 4-month surgical posting plus 4 months of a speciality. In the first year these tend to come in groups to complement each other. For example, a general medical posting, a surgical posting in orthopaedics and Accident and Emergency as a speciality, would constitute a complementary group. A & E links well with orthopaedics for obvious reasons.

In the second year there is more freedom of choice. Some specialities have a greater number of postings available than others, so the likelihood of you getting your choice of post is higher. Some specialities, unfortunately, have limited numbers. For example, Laboratory medicine or Microbiology may only have positions for one or two trainees every 4 months. General medicine, on the other hand, will have a far greater number of spaces available for every 4-month post. When you are considering what to choose we would advise putting posts with a higher probability of you getting your choice at the top of the list (e.g. General Medicine). This means you are less likely to get that one posting you're really trying to avoid! Be prepared for disappointment; it is unlikely that you'll get all three positions you wanted for that year.

If the unthinkable does happen and you get that one post you had really been dreading, don't panic. It's only 4 months of your life and it will fly by. Try not to dwell on your disappointment, but instead, draw on the positive things from the job that you will be able to use in the future. You will learn a great deal from *any* speciality that you spend time in. No matter how obscure the speciality or how far from your career choice it may be, it will have something to offer you.

You may dread that post in psychiatry, but you will come out with new and improved skills that you can continue to use in your career: the management of the acutely agitated patient and improved communication skills – vital in any speciality.

Draw the positives from your placement: aspects that you can use in any career and skills that will make you a better doctor all round. The posts allocated to you will not affect your application for speciality training, so don't worry if you are not given a 4-month post in your career-choice specialty.

Competencies

Certain objectives must be met in order to progress through your training. These are not there to make your life difficult, although it might seem like this sometimes, but they are there to ensure that you learn. There are a number of competencies that must be met and a document has been produced detailing these. This is available on the Modernising Medical Careers (MMC) Website (www.mmc.nhs.uk) for you to download. Various assessment methods will be used to demonstrate your ability in each competency. The competencies that must be met are listed below. They are based upon the GMC principles in 'good medical practice' (www.gmc-uk.org):

- Good clinical care
  - History, examination and record keeping skills
  - Appropriate time management and decision making
  - Understanding and applying the basis of good quality care and ensuring and promoting patient safety
  - Knowing and applying the principles of infection control
  - Understanding and applying the principles of health promotion and public health
  - Understanding and applying the principles of medical ethics and other legal issues
- Maintaining good medical practice
- Relationships with patients and communication
- Working with colleagues
- Teaching and training
- Professional behaviour and probity
- Acute care

Your ability in each competency will be demonstrated through various methods of assessment. An example of an assessment method is the Work Place Assessments (detailed later). There are a number to complete in year one and in year two. You will have to prove you are able to carry out and apply procedures with confidence, and have a colleague – anyone from the multidisciplinary team – to confirm this. Early completion of the work place assessments will demonstrate your understanding of the importance of time management and organization of paper work.

Methods of assessing the competencies may vary between deaneries. Other examples of assessment methods are given in Fig. 15.

Method of assessment	Description
Multi source feedback	A collective view of your performance as a doctor through the opinions of other health care professionals
	Can also be described as a mini-PAT (Peer Assessment Tool) or a TAB (Team Assessment of Behaviour)
Direct observation of the doctor	Mini clinical evaluation exercise (Mini-CEX) is an evaluation by a senior member of medical staff of a clinical situation you were involved in
	Direct observation of Practical Procedures (DOPS) is the assessment of a procedure carried out by yourself. The assessor can be any member of the multidisciplinary team (similar to work place assessments)
Case based discussion	Structured discussion of clinical cases managed by yourself. This encourages reflective practice and self evaluation

Fig. 15 Examples of assessment methods.

Teaching

Teaching is compulsory and you must attend a minimum number of teaching sessions to become registered with the GMC after your first year. You will need to sign in to teaching sessions as proof of attendance. Instead of trying to avoid these sessions, think positively; it gives you 2 hours every 2 weeks where you can escape the daily routines of the ward you are working in. There will be days where you'll be grateful that you can silence your bleeper! Also, try to organize a rota with your colleagues to ensure that everyone gets the chance to attend teaching. Finally, remember, there is much to be learned, and these lectures are actually most useful and worthwhile. For example, the teaching in your Deanery will cover a wide range of subjects – from your future career plans to clinical problems that you will commonly encounter in your daily practice.

E-portfolio

A portfolio containing information on what you have achieved in your daily work is required for registration and completion of both years. This can be completed on-line. Completion on-line saves a lot of time and paperwork, and by the time you read this it is likely that everyone will be completing the portfolio on-line.

The e-portfolio has a number of sections for you to complete. Examples are given below.

Presented evidence

EDUCATIONAL LOG

This contains details of all the educational activities you have undertaken, including teaching sessions attended and the time spent at these lectures, papers, tutorials, presentations, procedures, exams etc.

SIGNIFICANT EVENTS

Every 4 months you are required to complete either a multi-source feedback (MSF) or a significant event analysis (SEA) form. There will be one SEA in the first year and two in the second year. This is the minimum requirement and there is no limit to the number you can complete. See below for details.

PERSONAL DEVELOPMENT PLAN (PDP)

This looks at the ways in which you have been assessed, how you would judge your performance in the assessments, and what you would like to achieve or change in your next post. This should be filled out after each post so that you can set yourself achievable objectives.

Workplace assessment (WPA)

These are procedures that must be completed and signed off by a colleague as detailed in the competencies above. Your colleagues will be able to complete their assessment of you on-line, giving a score for each procedure completed satisfactorily. The assessor is someone with whom you are working. It can be anyone from the multidisciplinary team. For example, it would be appropriate for a member of the nursing staff to assess your ability to give an injection safely and correctly. You will need to take responsibility for achieving these competencies and will have to ask to be assessed by your colleagues. Sometimes it feels like the work place assessments interfere with your work and take up too much time. They are the last thing you have time to think about as a junior doctor. However, try not to leave them to the last minute, complete them early in each post and you will be under less stress later in the post.

Multi-source feedback (MSF)

Every alternate post, five MSF forms will need to be completed. Four of the multidisciplinary team you have worked with in a given post will complete evaluation forms on your performance in that position. You can choose who assesses you. There has to be a variety of people evaluating you: a consultant (alternatives are GPs and Staff Grades), a senior trainee (specialist registrar), a senior nurse (or practice nurse) and finally, anyone else of your choice (e.g. a pharmacist or a physiotherapist). You will also need to fill out an MSF form evaluating yourself.

In the past it was your responsibility to hand out forms to those you wished to assess you. Now it is much easier. Your colleagues can fill out an evaluation form on-line. All you need to do is advise them of the website address and provide them with your full name and GMC number. Once they have filled out the evaluation form they simply submit it. This eliminates the task of collecting the evaluation forms. Each Deanery is likely to have a specific time scale for requesting and submitting MSF forms.

Posts and meetings

This is where the meetings with your educational supervisor will be logged. You should aim to meet with them at the start of the post to sign an educational agreement. They will complete an evaluation of you at the end of the post, called the supervisor's report. You can see how well they have rated you in this section of the e-portfolio. In this section you can also see the scores that your colleagues have given you in the MSF evaluations.

Significant event analysis (SEA)

A significant event is an experience at work that has affected you in some way. It can be positive or negative as long as it is something you have learned from and that others can learn from.

A template is available on the e-portfolio. The SEA should contain the following:

- When did the event happen?
- What happened?
- Why did it happen?
- What have you learned?
- What have you changed?

One example of a significant event would be a drug error. There are a number of possibilities; the wrong drug was prescribed, the wrong dose was prescribed, the patient was given something they were known to be allergic to or the drug was prescribed but not given. For a SEA you need to look at the questions above, answer them truthfully and try to learn from the experience and change your practice if necessary.

The important point to make with relation to the SEA is not to look at it as a way of finding something negative in your abilities as a doctor. Remember, it doesn't have to be a negative, you can choose a positive event where the multidisciplinary team worked well together resulting in a positive outcome for the patient. Also it doesn't have to be about your practice alone but could be your team's practice.

Work experience and study leave

In the second year of training there is an opportunity to take time out of your current job in order to experience a 'taster' of the speciality you are interested in following as a career. So, although you may not have been allocated a posting in your career of choice, you will still have the opportunity to gain some experience in it. There is a time limit of around 5 days to these taster sessions. You will need permission from your tutor and from the people you are working with at the time, as you don't want to leave your colleagues struggling with their own work and yours in addition. There will also be work involved; it's not just an easy few days off! Firstly, you have to provide information to your tutor about what you will be doing, and be able to prove that it will be of value. After completion you will be expected to provide evidence outlining what you gained from the experience. This can be put in your portfolio. And don't forget, the taster session is something that you need to organize yourself.

Additional study days are available. The number of days may vary between Deaneries. Funding for study leave expenses may vary between Deaneries and some may not provide any funding. The only funding will be for essential courses undertaken in the 2 years (both ILS and ALS as mentioned below). As with the taster session, you will have to provide evidence of the educational value of the study leave, and it will only be granted with the approval of your educational supervisor.

Time is allocated specifically for the Immediate Life Support (ILS) and Advanced Life Support (ALS) courses. As part of your training you will be expected to complete both ILS and ALS courses. You cannot complete the first year without passing ILS and, equally, you cannot complete the second year without completing the ALS course. These courses are paid for by your Deanery.

Specialty exams

Although it is possible to take study leave it is important to mention that, as Foundation Year Doctors, you are strongly discouraged from doing specialty exams. The aim of Foundation Years is generic training and ongoing assessment, specialty exams should be taken once you have entered into specialty training. Passing the MRCP and MRCS exams from the old training system will not provide you with an advantage when applying for specialty training.

Feedback

In order for MMC to continue to improve and progress it is important that you provide your Deanery with your opinion on Foundation. It is vital that you complete the feedback forms for teaching sessions and the 'end of post' questionnaires. With the information you provide you can help to improve the posts you have worked in and make them a more enjoyable experience for your colleagues who follow.

Careers advice

During Foundation you will have the opportunity to discuss future career plans with your Foundation tutor. There is a specific section to complete for this in your portfolio. If you are finding it hard to make such a big decision in only 2 years then take the opportunity to arrange a couple of taster sessions. This may help. You may find the information below on fixed-term specialist training posts helpful if you are finding it difficult to make a career choice.

What to do if you are having problems

One of the differences between the Foundation Programme and the old job of Junior House Officer is the support that is available. If you are having problems in any aspect of your job seek help sooner rather than later. Your educational supervisor will be your first contact if there are problems in a specific post. If the problem is more generalized then your Foundation tutor would be the most appropriate person to contact. The online system of NHS Dots makes it easy to contact your tutor and your supervisor.

And after the foundation years?

More information is now available on Speciality Training, which will follow the first 2 years of training. However, this information is still limited. Any information we give you now is likely to change and will continue to change. Keep up to date with plans for Specialist Training posts on the Modernising Medical Careers Website (www.mmc.nhs.uk).

Application process

Fig. 16 shows a description of the type of posts you will be applying for.

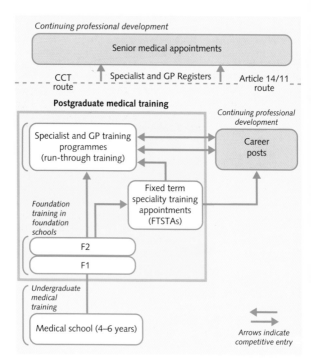

Fig. 16 UK MMC career framework. (Adapted from www.mimc.nhs.uk, with permission.)

Specialist and GP training (run-through training)

August 2007 will be the start date for the first entrants into Speciality Training. At the end of your foundation training you will apply for a run-through training programme in your chosen speciality. The run-through training posts will be structured around a curriculum with the aim of achieving a Certificate of Completion of Training (CCT) at the end the training. The length of the training post will depend on the speciality.

Fixed-term specialist training appointments (FTSTA)

Most people will apply for and aim to achieve a run-through training post. If you are unsuccessful in your application for run-through training there are other options. There will also be Fixed Term Training Posts in given specialities. These are likely to be 1 or 2 years in duration. They will provide similar training to the run-through posts but they do not offer progressive training. They will provide qualifications that will allow you to re-apply to enter run-through training at a later stage. FTSTAs will be a good alternative to run-through training for those of you who are not decided on a speciality.

Career posts

The final path that can be taken is a career post. This is MMC's equivalent to the current Staff Grade Post. These posts do not provide formal training with the end objective of a CCT; however, professional development and assessment will still be essential. You must have 3 years of postgraduate training to enter into a Career post.

Further information

There are a number of sources where you can obtain more detailed information:

- Modernising Medical Careers Website (www.mmc.nhs.uk)
- British Medical Association Website (www.bma.org.uk)
- General Medical Council Website (www.gmc-uk.org)

In addition to these sources remember that your tutors are also a great source of information. Talk to them, they are there to help.

Practical procedures

Practical procedures

Preparing a patient for a procedure

Laying a trolley

Laying a trolley is a vital skill. It should be performed meticulously to ensure a sterile field.

- Collect all the equipment you need for a given procedure. You will commonly need:
  - a dressing pack
  - a green (21G) needle to draw up lidocaine and to inject it into deeper tissue
  - an orange (27G) needle to administer local anaesthetic to the skin
  - 10 mL and 20 mL syringes
  - packets of gauze
  - iodine or chlorhexidine solution; check that your patient is not allergic to iodine
  - surgical tape
  - sterile gloves
  - sharps bin.
- Ask for help. You will need another pair of hands later.
- Place all the items except for the dressing pack on the bottom shelf of your trolley and take the trolley to the patient's bedside.
- Whatever procedure you are about to perform, tell the patient what you are going to do.
- Position the patient and yourself so that you are comfortable. Procedures always take longer than expected.
- Place an incontinence (inco) pad under the patient. This protects the bed and the patient from any blood and cleaning solution that you spill. The patient and nursing staff will thank you!
- Open the dressing pack with the tips of your fingers. Trying not to touch more than the corners, open the outer packaging. There will be another package inside, together with paper towels and a yellow bag. Take the yellow refuse bag and stick it on the end of the trolley.
- Peel open the orange needle package and drop the contents onto sterile paper without actually touching it. Repeat for all the other items you might need (needles, gloves, gauze, syringes, etc.).
- Wash your hands thoroughly. Dry them with paper towels and put on your gloves. Your hands are now sterile and you cannot touch anyone or anything that is not – this includes any part of the patient you have not cleaned with iodine or chlorhexidine.

Local anaesthetic

- Ask your assistant to pour the cleaning solution into the pot on your trolley.
- Clean the appropriate area on your patient using gauze or cotton wool. Apply the solution in a circular motion, working from the area outwards. Give yourself a large clean area. Do not go over where you have been with the same swab. Go over it again with a new swab if necessary. This area is now sterile and you can touch it. Cover any remaining part of the patient that is not sterile and which you might touch accidentally with drapes or the sterile sheet in the dressing pack.

- Ask your assistant to show you the bottle of local anaesthetic and to confirm its name, strength and expiry date.
- Draw up the lidocaine in a 10 mL syringe. The maximum dose of 1% lidocaine is 20 mL; for 2% lidocaine it is 10 mL.

Note: Never use lidocaine plus adrenaline when suturing extremities (fingers, toes and noses).

- Attach an orange needle and puncture the skin fairly superficially, into the dermis near the site you want to anaesthetize. Enter at 45°, aspirate back on the syringe to check that you are not in a blood vessel and inject 1–2 mL of lidocaine. A small 'bleb' will appear, allowing you to push the needle in further and deeper. Aspirate as you go and continue to inject the local anaesthetic along the line of the cut or where you will suture.
- Once you have injected superficially, remove the orange needle and replace it with a green one to anaesthetize more deeply, aspirating before you inject throughout. This time, ensure you inject 90° to the skin.
- Allow anaesthetic to work. The reason patients sometimes complain of pain after receiving local anaesthetic is often because the anaesthetic has not had time to work.

Suturing

There are many ways to suture (ask any surgeon) and the best way to learn is by watching and then doing. We will not go into further details here.

Finishing

When you have finished your procedure:

- Ensure all your sharps are thrown away. This is your responsibility alone.
- Clean the patient with normal saline and some clean swabs. Ensure all the cleaning solution and blood is cleaned off.
- Discard the inco pad.
- Put green drapes and gowns in the laundry basket. Ensure all other disposable items are cleaned up and put in your yellow bag. Throw this in the appropriate place and replace all other items. If you are lucky, your assistant will help, but don't assume this.

Venepuncture

Equipment

- Tourniquet • Gloves • Sharps box • Alcohol swab • Gauze or cotton wool
- Sticking plaster • Needle and syringe or vacutainer • Blood bottles

Method

- Tell the patient what you are about to do.
- Place the patient's arm on a pillow and make sure it is comfortable.
- Attach the tourniquet to the upper arm.
- Don your gloves.
- Examine and palpate for a vein in the antecubital fossa.
- Swab the skin with an alcohol swab and leave to dry.
- Insert the needle at 30° and advance until you feel the vein wall 'give' (Fig. 17).
- Attach the vacutainer tube, or gently pull back if using a syringe. (Note: For some samples, e.g. calcium, you need to take an uncuffed sample. Release the tourniquet when you have entered the vein).
- Remove the tourniquet if still attached.
- Withdraw the needle and syringe, simultaneously pressing down on the puncture with the gauze.
- Dispose of the needle immediately in the sharps box.
- Transfer blood to bottles if not using vacutainer.
- Apply sticking plaster.

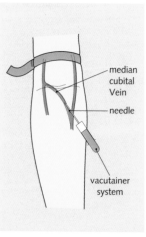

Fig. 17 Venepuncture.

median cubital Vein

needle

vacutainer system

> ## Notes
>
> Don't ask the patient to bend the arm up; this does not apply pressure to the puncture and will result in a bigger bruise

Difficult venepuncture

If you are having difficulty taking blood, abandon the vacutainer. The lack of a 'flashback' makes finding deep-seated veins hard and the vacuum can collapse small veins, especially in older people.

If neither antecubital fossa yields a vein, try the forearm, radial aspect of the wrists, back of the hand or even the base of the thumb. For these small veins, try a smaller needle (23G, blue – but no smaller than this) or a butterfly system.

If you still have trouble, consider using the feet – this is more painful.

As a last resort, or in an emergency when the peripheral circulation is shut down, consider a femoral stab:

- locate the femoral pulse
- swab the groin
- aim 1 cm medial to the femoral pulse, with the needle at right angles to the skin

Use of the femoral stab is a last resort – don't make it part of your phlebotomy routine!

Special groups

- IV drug users: if you can't get blood from an IV drug user, ask where the veins are (some will actually take the blood for you!).
- Patients with renal disease: any patient who is on dialysis or approaching the need for dialysis requires care in taking blood.
- Never perform venepuncture on a limb with an AV fistula (unless the renal team tell you that it's OK). Do not use veins at the wrist or forearm in either limb; these are vital for future fistula creation. Use the antecubital veins or veins on the back of the hand.

Cannulation

Equipment

- Tourniquet • Gloves • Sharps box • Alcohol swab • Gauze or cotton wool
- 5 mL syringe with saline • Cannula • Vecafix

Method

- Tell the patient who you are and what you are going to do.
- Attach the tourniquet to the upper arm.
- Examine and palpate the arm for a vein. Look at:
    - the back of the hand – this is a common site but can be fragile and mobile in the elderly
    - the antecubital fossa will always have a vein but might be uncomfortable for the patient
    - the anatomical snuffbox at wrist – 'houseman's friend'.
- Swab the selected vein.
- Anchor the vein and insert the cannula at 30° to the skin (Fig. 18), advance until you feel give in the vein wall.
- Watch for flashback at the base of the cannula.
- Pull the needle part of the cannula (the stylet) back 1–2 mm and watch blood flow into the plastic tubing.
- Slide the needle back while advancing the cannula into the vein.
- Remove the needle completely and place the cap on the end of the cannula.
- Dispose of the needle immediately. Tape down using Vecafix.
- Flush through with 5 mL normal saline.

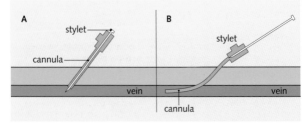

Fig. 18 Cannulation of a vein. Ensure that the stylet and cannula have entered the vein (A) before withdrawing the stylet and advancing the cannula (B).

Hints and tips

Finding the vein is the most important part of the exercise. If you have problems, try the following:

After putting on tourniquet, ask patient to drop the hand by the side and to clench and unclench the fist. Do something else in the meantime, e.g. draw-up your saline, open up the cannula

If you cannot feel a vein in one arm, do not attempt to go in blind – stop and review the other arm

If still have no luck, ask the patient to put both hands in some warm water to help vasodilation

If really desperate, try sticking GTN patches to the antecubital fossa veins

Foot veins are sometimes used, but this can be painful for the patient and should only be used as last resort

Special groups

The reservations made about groups such as IV drug abusers and renal patients in the Venepuncture section also apply here.

Cannula sizes

Fig. 19 outlines the different sizes, colours and uses of some common cannulas.

Some common cannulas			
Colour	Size	Flow rate	Uses
Blue	22G	36 mL/min	In children and patients with difficult small veins, e.g. elderly. Only use for infusions such as N saline, standard antibiotics and heparin
Pink	20G	61 mL/min	Standard sizes for routine use. Useful for most infusions and blood. 18G better for transfusions
Green	18G	90 mL/min	
White	17G	140 mL/min	Not very commonly but useful in patients who need large amounts of IV fluid or for blood transfusions
Grey	16G	200 mL/min	Used for patients in shock, e.g. GI bleeds, trauma situations. Also used for peripheral administration of certain drugs, e.g. amiodarone, dopamine/dobutamine
Brown	14G	300 mL/min	

Fig. 19 Examples of some common cannulas and their uses.

Arterial blood gas (ABG) measurement

Equipment

- ABG syringe (almost always preheparinized nowadays) • Alcohol swab • Gloves
- Sharps box • Gauze or cotton wool • Adhesive tape • 27G (orange) needle

Method

- Tell the patient what you are about to do.
- Palpate the site to be sampled. In general, the radial artery is best: it is most accessible, less susceptible to venous sampling and easiest to clean (see below).
- Swab the skin.
- Discard the needle from the ABG pack and attach a 27G needle (orange). This is much less painful, obviating the need for local anaesthetic.
- Hold the syringe like a pencil and enter the skin over the site of the palpated pulse, aiming proximally at an angle of 30° to the vertical (Fig. 20).
- Advance slowly along the line of the artery until you see a 'flashback'. If you fail to see a flashback, withdraw the needle slowly. Try palpating the artery again.
- Hold the syringe steady and allow the syringe to fill. You might need to draw back gently on the plunger if using a small needle.
- Once you have 0.5 mL of blood, withdraw the syringe and press firmly over the puncture site with a gauze swab for 2–3 min. Attach the gauze swab tightly to the skin with tape.

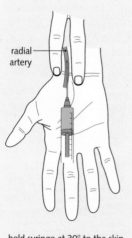

Fig. 20 Radial artery sampling. Use one hand to feel the radial pulse and insert the syringe at 30° to the skin surface.

radial artery

hold syringe at 30° to the skin

- Take the needle off the syringe and dispose of it. Carefully expel any air from the syringe (some packs have a filter that you can attach to the syringe to help with this).
- Cap the syringe with the cap provided and tip upside down a few times to mix well.
- Take the sample to the blood gas machine yourself or, if it needs to be sent to the biochemistry lab, place the sample in a plastic bag with a few ice cubes. Don't forget to put a label on the syringe.

Note: If you don't know how to use the blood gas analyser, ask someone. They cost thousands of pounds and a broken machine is extremely inconvenient.

Pitfalls

Unable to obtain blood: try a larger needle (blue or green); unless it is an emergency, you will have to inject local anaesthetic around the artery (be very careful to aspirate before injecting so as to avoid injecting lidocaine into the artery. A larger needle usually allows the blood gas syringe to fill without pulling back due to the arterial pressure.

Venous sampling: you might suspect this if the sample looks rather darker than expected. Samples from hypoxic patients may well be dark, however; a better guide is if the pO_2 or SaO_2 are much lower than the pulse oximetry readings – this suggests venous sampling.

Other sites

If you cannot get a radial artery sample, try a femoral artery sample:

- Use a standard 21G (green) needle; this is long enough to get to the femoral artery.
- Palpate the femoral pulse. In obese individuals, ask the patient to externally rotate the hip – this brings the artery closer to the surface.
- Clean the skin thoroughly.
- Place a finger on either side of the femoral pulse and insert the needle between the fingers, perpendicular to the skin. Beware – it is easy to give yourself a needlestick injury here.
- Advance until flashback occurs and syringe starts to fill.

If neither the radial or femoral artery site yields a sample, you could try a brachial sample. The technique is similar to the two above but the artery is often hard to find and can be quite mobile; this technique is also more uncomfortable for the patient. Try to use a 27G (orange) needle and consider using local anaesthetic.

If you can't get a sample after two or three attempts, call your senior.

Urinary catheterization – male

Equipment

- Urinary catheters – male or female length, sizes 12–16 ● Catheter dressing pack ● Sterile gloves ● Lidocaine gel ● 10 mL saline in a syringe ● Urometer or urine collection bag ● Saline for cleaning ● Kidney bowl

Method

- Tell the patient what you are about to do.
- Open all of the necessary equipment on your trolley.
- Place a clean drape around the patient's penis.
- Retract the foreskin and clean the glans thoroughly with saline.
- Coat the end of the catheter with lidocaine jelly. Insert the nozzle of the lidocaine gel gently into the preputial orifice and squeeze.
- Give the gel time to work (a few minutes).
- Place the kidney bowl on the bed between the patient's legs.
- Gently insert the catheter tip and advance. You might need to twist the catheter gently from side to side. Drape the other end of the catheter into the kidney bowl to catch any urine spillage.
- Push the catheter all the way in, even if urine starts to flow before it is fully inserted.
- Inflate the retaining balloon with 10 mL of saline.
- Carefully replace foreskin.
- Attach a bag or urometer.

Potential problems

Urine doesn't flow: either the bladder is empty or you are in a false passage. You can try a 50 mL flush of saline using a bladder syringe. If this can be introduced and withdrawn, you are likely to be in the bladder

Catheter won't pass: try a bigger catheter. This sounds paradoxical but a bigger catheter is stiffer and thus might negotiate a stricture or enlarged prostate. Make sure that the lidocaine gel has had long enough to work. If passing the catheter is painful, the perineal muscles will go into spasm, making passage of the catheter much more difficult

Blood in the urine: a small amount of blood in the urine or around the penile orifice indicates trauma inserting the catheter. If clots or dark blood are present in the urine, consider a three-way catheter to allow for irrigation

If you are still having problems, talk to a urologist. A suprapubic catheter is sometimes required but urologists have a number of other tricks that are useful for passing catheters!

Urinary catheterization – female

Equipment

• Urinary catheters – male or female length, sizes 12–16 • Catheter dressing pack • Sterile gloves • Lidocaine gel • 10 mL saline in a syringe • Urometer or urine collection bag • Saline for cleaning • Kidney bowl

Method

If you are asked to do this, it is usually because the nursing staff are having difficulty. This means that you too are likely to have difficulty!

- Tell the patient what you are going to do.
- Ensure that the perineum is well lit.
- Abduct the legs as far as possible.
- Ask an assistant to hold folds of abdominal fat out of the way if necessary.
- Look carefully to distinguish the urethral orifice from the vagina (Fig. 21).
- If in doubt as to the position of the catheter (i.e. if no urine flows), flush and withdraw 50 mL of saline.

Fig. 21 Female catheterization.

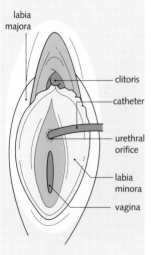

labia majora
clitoris
catheter
urethral orifice
labia minora
vagina

SC and IM injections

SC method

- Explain to the patient what you are about to do.
- Don gloves and draw up the medication to be given using the 21G (green) needle. Expel air from the syringe and attach the 27G needle.
- Swab the skin into a fold in a suitable site, e.g. forearm, triceps area, abdomen. Pinch the skin gently into a fold.
- Insert the needle horizontally into the fold of skin (Fig. 22).
- Draw back on the needle to ensure that you are not in a vein.
- Slowly inject the medication. Withdraw the needle and wipe the area with cotton wool.

IM method

- Explain to the patient what you are about to do.
- Don gloves and draw up the medication to be given using the 21G (green) needle. Expel air from the syringe and attach the 21G or 23G needle.

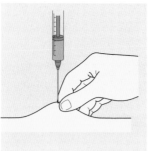

Fig. 22 Subcutaneous injection. Pinch a fold of skin between the thumb and forefinger, then inject into the fold.

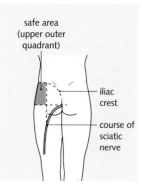

Fig. 23 The site for intramuscular injection.

safe area
(upper outer
quadrant)

iliac crest

course of sciatic nerve

- Swab the area to be injected – upper outer quadrant of buttock, deltoid area (Fig. 23), lateral thigh.
- Insert the needle to full depth perpendicular to the skin.
- Draw back on the needle to ensure it is not in a vein.
- Slowly inject the medication. If the patient complains of discomfort, stop for a few seconds until the pain eases, then continue more slowly.
- Withdraw the needle and wipe the area with cotton wool.

Hints

In obese individuals, a 21G needle will be needed, especially if injecting the buttock, in order to get as deep as the muscle layer. Injection into subcutaneous fat leads to poor absorption and occasionally to inflammation of the fat

At some time, you will be asked to perform IM injection in a confused, disturbed individual – often with the aim of sedation. This is permissible under common law, as long as you satisfy yourself that the patient is incapable of informed consent and that your actions are in the best interests of the patient. Think carefully before administering IM sedation to a confused patient who is wandering at night – ask yourself if you have been asked to do it because the nursing staff want a quiet night shift!

If you do administer sedation to a disturbed patient, ensure that you put your own safety first. A flailing arm plus a contaminated needle is a recipe for a needlestick injury and possible blood-borne infection. Get someone to help you, perhaps by gently restraining flailing arms, or by talking to distract the patient

ECGs and cardiac monitors

Equipment

• ECG machine • Adhesive electrodes • Razor

Method

- Explain to the patient what you are about to do.
- Attach the electrodes to the skin in the positions shown (Fig. 24). You will need to shave hairy areas to get a good contact. Note that accurate placement is important; having the chest leads in the wrong place can lead to an anterior MI being diagnosed as an inferior MI!
- Switch on the ECG machine. Ensure that the mains lead does not cross the electrode leads.
- Enter the patient details if required.
- Make sure that the FILTER button is on.
- Take the ECG (usually by pressing a button marked '12' or 'auto').

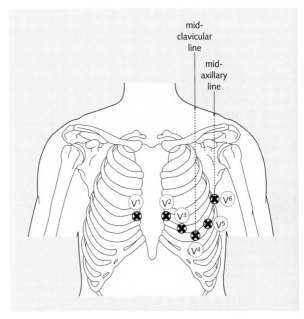

Fig. 24 Placement of ECG chest leads.

Pitfalls

Missing tracings: check all the lead attachments and replace any electrodes that are not adhering well. Twist the leads within the attaching clips to ensure that the leads are not pulling the adhesive pads off the patient

Wandering baseline/irregular baseline: repeat the tracing, asking the patient to relax and stay still. If this fails, attach the limb leads to the shoulders and hips; this cuts down on interference from limb muscle electrical signals

Interference on baseline: ensure no mains cables are crossing the ECG wires. If you still have a problem, try and run the ECG machine on its battery rather than on the mains. Still got a problem? Move the ECG machine to the other side of the bed and unplug any non-essential electrical equipment around the bed

Odd axis on ECG: make sure that you have the leads attached to the correct electrodes, especially the limb leads

If all else fails, get another machine

Lumbar puncture

Equipment

- Sterile gloves • Dressing pack • 1% or 2% lidocaine • Spinal needle – black (22G) is best, preferably with a round tip • Cleaning solution (iodine or chlorhexidine) • Gauze swabs • Micropore • Manometer and three-way tap • Three sterile specimen bottles • One glucose (oxalate – grey-topped) blood tube

Method

The most important thing to do is to position the patient correctly. Lay the patient on the left side, with the back parallel to the bed.

- Ask the patient to maximally flex the back to open up the spinous processes. Ensure the shoulders are square to the hips.
- Make sure the patient's back is straight and that you can feel the gaps between the spinous processes (Fig. 25).
- Feel the iliac crests and draw across the back to the other iliac crest.
- Feel down the spinous processes until you feel a gap as close to the vertical line you have drawn as you can. This is L3–L4.
- Choose the L3–L4 space or go a space higher to L2–L3.
- Get a chair. Sit down where you will perform the procedure. Raise the bed so you are comfortable.
- Set up your trolley:
  - label three specimen bottles: 1, 2, 3
  - prepare your trolley
  - wash your hands thoroughly.

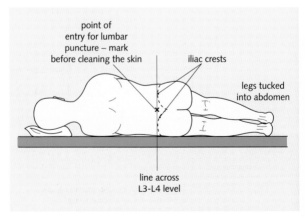

Fig. 25 Positioning of the patient for lumbar puncture. (Adapted from Sprigings D, Chambers J, Jeffrey A. *Acute Medicine*, 2nd edition, 1995 Blackwell Science.)

- Open up the three-way tap and manometer. Connect up and be certain you know which tap opens to the manometer and closes all the others, and then close it to the manometer and open to the 'outside world'.
- Check that the stylet passes through the needle properly.
- Clean over L2, L3 and L4, giving yourself a large area to work with. Drape your greens and administer local anaesthetic at L3–L4.
- Place the spinal needle over the site of lidocaine administration, bevel uppermost, and advance. Make sure the needle remains at 90° to the skin in all planes.
- Push through several layers of tissue (Fig. 26) until you feel the needle 'give'. Carefully remove the stylet 1–2 cm to see if you have clear CSF.
- Hold the end of the needle carefully but firmly with your left hand and pull the stylet out with your right – cover the end of the needle with your left thumb to prevent CSF leak.
- Attach the manometer with the three-way tap turned to allow CSF to go straight up. Measure the CSF pressure – it is in cmH$_2$O. Anything < 20 is normal. Give it time, especially with a small needle.
- Once the pressure is measured, you can collect CSF by turning tap so the spinal needle is open to you but the manometer is closed, retaining its column of fluid. Have bottle 1 ready and collect 10–12 drops of CSF. Put your thumb over the end and have your assistant take bottle 1 away and pass you bottle 2. Repeat with all three bottles.
- For the glucose sample, collect the column of CSF in the manometer by closing the spinal needle and opening the manometer to you. Beware – this comes out very fast.

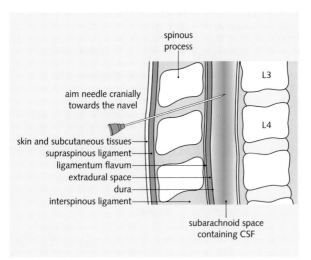

spinous process

L3

aim needle cranially towards the navel

L4

skin and subcutaneous tissues ——
supraspinous ligament ——
ligamentum flavum ——
extradural space ——
dura ——
interspinous ligament ——

subarachnoid space containing CSF

Fig. 26 Insertion of the lumbar puncture needle.

- Remove the manometer, put your thumb over the end of the spinal needle to prevent CSF loss before replacing the stylet; then remove the entire needle.
- Clean the patient's back and put a small dressing/plaster over the needle site. Move the patient back onto the back and advise rest for 1 h – local policy might advise differently on this time and can be up to 4 h. Check with your hospital policy.
- Send bottles 1 and 3 for cell count; this will differentiate a bloody tap from blood in the CSF. Send bottle 2 for biochemistry and xanthochromia.

Hints and tips

If you cannot get into the epidural space, make sure you are at 90 degrees to the skin in all planes. Sometimes you will find you have aimed skywards

If you still have no success or hit bone, go up a space to L2–L3

If you still have no success, sit the patient upright to perform the procedure. Again, mark out landmarks using the iliac crests and aim the needle at 90°. You cannot measure the pressure but will get your samples using this method

---

Nasogastric (NG) tubes

Equipment

- Gloves • NG tube • Litmus paper • KY jelly • Glass of water

Method

Usually, nurses manage to do this with no problems. It is unusual for them to call you. If they do:

- Tell the patient what you are going to do.
- Sit the patient upright.
- Cover the end of the tube lightly with lubricating jelly.
- Insert the tube into one nostril horizontally, and pass it down slowly.
- Ask the patient to start swallowing, and push the NG tube more quickly down. If the patient starts to choke, stop immediately. A glass of water can help them swallow, although most patients you want to place an NG tube in will either be unsafe to swallow water or will be nil by mouth!
- The patient should swallow the tube down. Check the position. There are differing local policies regarding checking NG tube positioning. Check what they are. They include:
  - aspirating slowly on the end of the NG tube and checking the secretions with litmus paper
  - injecting 20 mL of air and auscultating for 'bubbling' over the stomach
  - performing a chest X-ray to confirm the position. Specify on the X-ray request that it is for NG tube positioning because the X-ray used is of different penetration to highlight the tube.
- On the chest X-ray, look for the NG sitting in or towards the stomach bubble, beneath the diaphragm. If it deviates to the right or, less commonly, the left, it is in a bronchus and needs to be removed and re-sited.

Note: Do not attempt to pass an NG tube if there is any possibility of a skull fracture, e.g. CSF from the ear. A skull X-ray might be helpful, although this will not exclude a base of skull fracture.

Pleural tap

Equipment

- 1% or 2% lidocaine • Basic dressing pack with sterile towels • Sterile gloves
- Iodine- or chlorhexidine-based antiseptic • Sterile universal containers • 21G (green) needles • 27G (orange) needles • 16G (grey) cannula • 10 mL syringe • 20 mL syringe • An assistant

Method

- Explain to the patient what you are about to do.
- Sit the patient on the edge of the bed, arms folded in front of the body and leaning forward across a hospital table (Fig. 27).
- Before donning your gloves, check the site of the effusion on the chest X-ray and percuss down the chest. Place a cross on the lateral posterior aspect of the

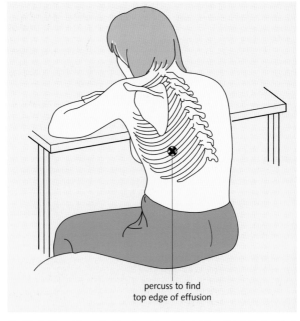

percuss to find
top edge of effusion

Fig. 27 Position of the patient for pleural tap. (Adapted from McLatchie G. *Oxford Handbook of Clinical Surgery*, 1st edition, 1990, by permission of Oxford University Press.)

chest, 3–5 cm below the level at which you can first percuss the effusion. Your cross should be in an intercostal space, over the top surface of a rib.

- Do not proceed if you cannot confidently percuss the effusion; get an ultrasound scan to mark the position.
- Don your gloves, place sterile towels below the target area and clean the skin with antiseptic.
- Draw up 5–10 mL of lidocaine and raise a bleb under the skin with a 27G needle.
- Infiltrate local anaesthetic using a 21G needle, slowly working down perpendicular to the skin. Aim over the top surface of the rib, pulling back before injecting anaesthetic. Stop when you aspirate fluid (Fig. 28).
- For a diagnostic tap, attach a fresh 21G needle to a 20 mL syringe, insert along the anaesthetized track at right angles to the skin and advance while at the same time pulling the plunger back. When fluid is first aspirated, stop – do not advance any further – and pull the plunger back until the syringe is full. Withdraw the needle and press over the site with gauze.
- For a therapeutic tap, attach a 50 mL Luer-lock syringe to a three-way tap. Attach a length of tubing to the side port of the three-way tap (a giving set works reasonably well). Put the other end of the tubing in a large sterile jug.
- Insert a 16G cannula along the anaesthetized track at right angles to the skin. When you see a fluid flashback, advance the cannula a little further, then push the plastic cannula as far into the thorax as it will go, keeping the stylet still. As you withdraw the stylet, put a thumb over the end of the cannula – this prevents a pneumothorax. If possible, ask the patient to breathe out and hold the breath in expiration as you withdraw the stylet.
- Attach the three-way tap to the cannula, ensuring that the cannula does not kink. You can now either allow the fluid to drain under gravity, or you can withdraw 50 mL using the syringe, then turn the three-way tap, and expel the contents of the syringe into the tubing.
- Once you have drained 1–1.5 L of fluid, remove the cannula and attached equipment and press over the hole with gauze for a minute.

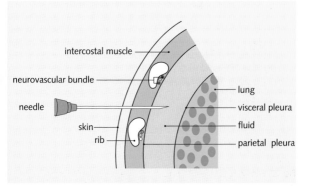

Fig. 28 Insertion of the needle for pleural tap.

Pitfalls

No fluid aspirated: try angling the needle down a little, to the side a little, or withdraw the needle a little. If you still fail to aspirate fluid, start again by percussing out the level of the effusion again. If you still cannot aspirate fluid, give up and request an ultrasound scan to locate the effusion

The patient is obese: for a diagnostic tap, try using a 16G or 18G cannula, or a 21G lumbar puncture needle; they are longer than a standard 21G needle. For a therapeutic tap, try using a long 14G cannula, or even better a cannula over stylet central line – rare, but very useful if you can find one!

Blood is aspirated: a small flash of blood is not unusual; this is caused by nicking blood vessels in the skin. Red fluid is either blood or a bloody effusion; put a little in a dish and see if it clots. If it doesn't clot, it is likely to be a bloody effusion. If it does clot, get out and seek help

The flow rate slows down during aspiration: some effusions, especially malignant effusions with a high protein content, can be very viscous. This can result in the cannula becoming narrowed during aspiration, which leads to difficulty aspirating fluid. You might need to use a new cannula

The patient is uncomfortable: if the discomfort occurs on inserting the needle, more local anaesthetic is needed. If cough or discomfort occurs during a therapeutic aspiration, this suggests that the lung has re-expanded and the visceral pleural is in contact with the needle. Stop the aspiration if this occurs

The patient becomes unwell: vasovagal reactions are not uncommon during pleural taps; if the patient feels faint, stop, withdraw the needle immediately, and lie the patient down. Adequate local anaesthetic can help to avoid this. Less commonly, the shift of the lung and mediastinum can lead to changes in autonomic tone, or to circulatory collapse. Do not aspirate more than 1–1.5 L of fluid in a single sitting

Sending the fluid

Send the fluid off for microscopy, culture and sensitivity, for cytology, and for protein and LDH levels. If TB is at all possible, request acid-fast staining. If the effusion accompanies a pneumonia, place some of the fluid on ice and request the pH of the fluid – this is vital for deciding whether a chest drain is required.

What to do afterwards

Order a chest X-ray, even after a diagnostic or failed tap, to check for pneumothorax. A small pneumothorax does not need aspirating but might require another X-ray in a few hours to ensure that it is not increasing in size. Write a brief note in the patient notes regarding the procedure.

Giving IV drugs and fluids

Equipment

• IV fluids • Giving set • Cannula • Syringe driver/pump

Method

You might be asked to give drugs IV. This could be as simple as giving an IV bolus through a cannula or giving drugs through a drip. Make sure that you read the instructions provided carefully:

• Ensure that the cannula is in place and flushes easily with saline.
• Make sure you know what infusion rate the drug should be injected at – slow bolus through a big vein protects the veins and prevents the cannula from tissuing.

If the drug is diluted in solution (50–500 mL normal saline) or you are asked to put a bag of fluid up on a patient:

• Put the bag of fluid up on a drip stand.
• Connect one end of the giving set to the bag and close the valve in the plastic tubing.
• Squeeze the reservoir so it is half filled with fluid and the remainder drips in.
• Open the valve and let the remainder of the fluid run through so no air bubbles remain. Once there are no air pockets and fluid runs freely out of the end of the giving set, attach to the end of the cannula.
• Set the drip rate or put tubing through the fluid pump.

Always ask another person to check the drugs you are administering. Ask them to confirm the drug name, dose, method of delivery and expiry date. This includes any additives e.g. KCl.

Always check you have the right patient – check the wristband for identification.

Remember that some drugs need to be administered with care, e.g. vancomycin must be given as a slow infusion; Pabrinex and vitamin K are dangerous if given as a fast bolus. Some drugs are irritant and will need larger veins; the cannula should be well flushed after administering such drugs.

Ascitic tap and/or drainage (Paracentesis)

Equipment

• Dressing pack • Lots of gauze swabs • Sterile gloves • Iodine/cleaning solution • 10 mL syringe • 50 mL syringe • Green and orange needle • 1% or 2% lidocaine • Ascitic drain and bag • Scalpel • Adhesive dressing

Method

- Explain to the patient what you are going to do.
- Expose the patient's abdomen fully and percuss out ascitic fluid. Demonstrate shifting dullness or a fluid thrill. Percuss either right or left iliac fossa – this is where you will insert the drain. Mark it with a pen if necessary.
- Prepare yourself and your trolley:
  - wash your hands
  - open up your dressing pack
  - pour iodine into a pot
  - put on sterile gloves.
- Draw up the lidocaine using the green needle. Replace the green needle with the orange needle and fill this too.
- Have your helper open the ascitic drain and bag for you. The ascitic drain is usually a small-bore tube with an introducer inside. It is inserted like an IV cannula. Familiarize yourself with it before proceeding.
- Prepare the skin and inject local anaesthetic with the orange and then the green needle. You will finally feel a give, then aspirate straw-coloured ascitic fluid easily. Withdraw the needle slightly and inject more local anaesthetic.
- Remove the needle and nick the skin over the local anaesthetic with a scalpel.
- Take the ascitic drain, with a 20 or 50 mL syringe attached, and enter the skin at 90 degrees, pushing gently until ascitic fluid is again aspirated. Now, as with a cannula, slowly withdraw the introducer while at the same time advancing the drain until it is inserted (Fig. 29).

Pitfalls

No aspiration: you are in the wrong place. Repercuss and try again. If you are still unsuccessful then you might need an ultrasound to mark a spot for you
No drainage: think of the following:

  • blockage – try flushing drain with sterile saline
  • kink in the tube – check where tube is tied in and ensure it is not kinked
  • drain has fallen out – remove the drain and, if necessary, replace with new drain at new site

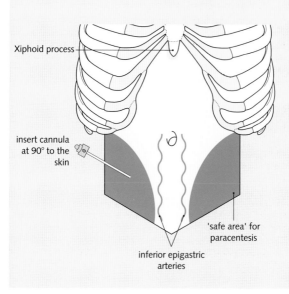

Xiphoid process

insert cannula at 90° to the skin

'safe area' for paracentesis

inferior epigastric arteries

Fig. 29 Ascitic tap.

- Remove the introducer completely and attach it to the drainage bag. Clamp it when 1 L has been drained. Large-volume paracentesis can be carried out as a therapeutic measure if accompanied by intravenous volume replacement, e.g. with 1 unit of 20% albumin for each 2 L drained. Check with your seniors.
- Suture the drain in place and cover it with an adhesive dressing. Clean the patient of remaining iodine with saline.

Simple aspiration

Diagnostic aspirations should be performed with the same care as insertion of a drain. They are simple in that they can be performed with a green needle. Enough fluid should be taken for culture (M, C and S), protein, glucose and αFP.

Chest drain insertion

Equipment

- Drapes • Suture kit • Dressing pack • Gauze • Scalpel • 1% or 2% lidocaine
- 2/0 silk suture on curved needle • 10 mL syringe • Orange and green needle
- Sterile gloves • Iodine/cleaning agent • Chest drain (Seldinger or 'trochar')
- Chest drain bag (for pleural effusion) or water-tight bottle containing some normal saline or sterile water (for pneumothorax) • An assistant

Method

- Tell the patient what you are going to do.
- Confirm the position of the pneumothorax/effusion clinically and also with a chest X-ray.
- Sit the patient upright, legs over the side of bed, leaning over a high table so the arms are up, the back is straight and you have access to the affected side of the chest. In an unwell patient you might have to perform this with the patient at 45 degrees.
- Prepare the underwater seal – fill a bottle one-third with sterile water. The end of the tube should be 2–3 cm into the water.
- Choose the chest drain; tailor it to the patient by looking at how much rib space is available. Seldinger chest drains are used much more frequently. Traditional 'trochar' drains are increasingly becoming the remit of specialist chest teams. Seldinger drains are much less traumatic for both patients and doctors alike. Some chest physicians however still prefer larger drains, particularly for effusions and empyemas – as a guide 24F is suitable for a pneumothorax; use 28–32F for effusions and empyemas.
- Don your gloves and prepare your trolley so that all the items are within easy reach.
- Prepare the patient's skin with chlorhexidine or iodine and perform pleural aspiration in the mid-axillary line at the 4th–5th intercostal space; aim above the rib.
- Once pleural fluid has been located, insert more local anaesthetic – be generous. Use up to 15 mL in the area around the aspiration site. Some patients might find this uncomfortable, so you can give a small dose of diamorphine IV with 10 mg metoclopramide IV.

SELDINGER TECHNIQUE
This technique is virtually identical to that of inserting an ascitic drain or central line.

- Take the large-bore needle provided in the chest drain pack and attach a 10 or 20 mL syringe containing a small amount of the local anaesthetic. Re-insert the needle over the previous aspiration site at 90° to the skin. Introduce the needle until pleural fluid can readily be aspirated.
- Remove the syringe, keeping the needle very still and immediately put your thumb over the end of the needle.

- Take the guidewire provided and insert through the end of the needle, and advance until about two-thirds of the wire is inserted. The wire should advance freely and should not be forced.

- Holding the wire, remove the needle, keeping the wire in place. Make a nick with a scalpel where the wire enters the skin. Insert the dilator over the wire and then remove.

- Insert the drain over the wire. Keep one hand over the wire at all times. When the drain has been inserted, slowly withdraw the wire from the drain while advancing the drain further. Remove the wire completely and immediately place a thumb over the end of the drain to prevent fluid leakage or the introduction of air into the pleural space.

- Connect the end of the drain to an underwater seal.

TRADITIONAL 'TROCHAR' TECHNIQUE

- Make a 1–2 cm incision with the scalpel in line with the ribs, remaining just above the lower rib. Once through skin and into subcutaneous fat, blunt-dissect down with forceps. Continue until you reach the pleura. This can be painful, so have remaining local anaesthetic to hand and inject into pleura if necessary.

- Take the introducer out of the chest drain, so only the tubing remains. Once you have blunt-dissected the pleura and fluid or air begins to escape, insert the drain into the hole. It should enter the pleural cavity easily, but keep a finger over the end of the drain until it is connected to the bag or underwater seal.

SECURING THE DRAIN

- Place a 1-mattress suture on either side of drain and pull taut. Place another suture in the middle of incision around the drain. Tie the two side sutures, so the skin is pulled tight, then secure around the drain by coiling round several times. Leave the central suture free, to be tied when the drain is removed.

- Place pads of gauze around drain and secure with dressing. Secure the proximal part of the drain to the patient with tape.

- Ensure that the drain is draining/bubbling freely. Get a post-procedure chest X-ray to review the position.

Underwater seals

Underwater seals are used to drain air from the pleural cavity. They are always kept below the level of the chest. When the pressure of air in the pleural cavity rises, air is forced from the chest into the water, and it bubbles. Normal respiration causes some movement in air pressure and the water level oscillates accordingly – this is known as 'swinging'. If the fluid level does not swing, it means the tube is:

- blocked – flushing it might help, or it might need to be replaced
- kinked – the dressing needs to be removed and the tube reviewed
- in the wrong place – it was inserted incorrectly or has fallen out; a chest X-ray will confirm.

If there is no bubbling but the tube is still swinging, the pneumothorax has probably been corrected. If this is confirmed by chest X-ray the drain can be removed, after 24 h.

If there is continuous bubbling and no or only partial resolution of the pneumothorax on chest X-ray, then there is a continuous leak and a chest physician/thoracic surgeon should be contacted.

Chest drain removal

Once the mattress sutures are in place, removal of the drain is straightforward.

Equipment

• Dressing pack • Sterile scissors • Sterile gauze • Chlorhexidine/Iodine for cleaning

Method

- Remove dressings from around the drain.
- Clean the whole area with iodine/chlorhexidine.
- Cut free the ties to the drain from side sutures but do not untie the sutures holding the skin together.
- Ask the patient to breathe in deeply and exhale fully. Get your assistant to pull the drain out while you pull the central suture tight closed.
- Tie the suture. Clean and dress the area.
- Repeat the chest X-ray.
- Remove sutures at 1 week.

Central line placement

Equipment

• Central line dressing pack with gown and drapes • Sterile gloves • Iodine or chlorhexidine antiseptic 1% or 2% lidocaine • Central line (preferably at least a triple lumen line) • Saline or heparin saline to flush line • Stitch and stitch holders • Scissors • Scalpel blade • 21G (green) and 27G (orange) needles • 2 × 10 mL syringes • Occlusive dressing • An assistant

Method

- Explain to the patient what you are about to do.

- Choose the site for insertion; jugular or femoral carry less bleeding risk and low risk of pneumothorax; subclavian is a cleaner site and is technically more difficult; we have not covered the technique here. Small ultrasound machines are increasingly being used to correctly identify the internal jugular vein. Training in their use is usually available in your local Trust. For drug administration, IV access and even emergency pacing, femoral is probably the easiest site.

- Don your gloves and gown, clean and drape the site.

- Tilt the head end of the bed down by 10–15°.

- Draw up 10 mL of lidocaine; raise a bleb on the skin with a 27G needle.

- Infiltrate local anaesthetic all around the site, working down towards the vein. Pull back on the plunger before injecting each time to ensure that you don't inject into the vein.

- Have the assistant open the central line pack and take all the items out. Ensure that the wire moves freely on its reel – you will need to advance the wire one-handed.

- Flush each port of the central line with saline or heparin saline, and close off each line except the distal (usually brown) line; the wire threads through this line.

- Attach a syringe to the large needle provided:
  - right femoral line: find the arterial pulse and enter the skin 1 cm medial to this, at 45° to the vertical and heading parallel to the artery. Advance slowly, aspirating all the time, until you enter the vein (Fig. 30)
  - right jugular line: palpate the carotid artery with your left hand, covering the artery with your fingers. Insert the needle 0.5–1 cm laterally to the artery, aiming at 45° to the vertical. In men, aim for the right nipple; in women, aim for the iliac crest. Advance slowly, aspirating all the time, until you enter the vein (Fig. 31). If you fail to aspirate blood after entering 3–4 cm, withdraw, re-enter at the same point but aim slightly more medially.

- Once the needle is in the vein, ensure that you can reliably aspirate blood. Remove the syringe, keeping the needle very still, and immediately put your thumb over the end of the needle.

- Insert the wire into the end of the needle, and advance the wire until at least 30 cm are inserted. The wire should advance very easily – do not force it.

Fig. 30 Femoral artery sampling.

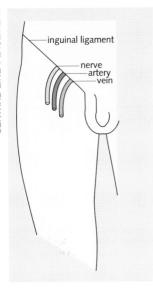

inguinal ligament

nerve
artery
vein

- Keeping one hand on the wire at all times, remove the needle, keeping the wire in place. Make a nick in the skin where the wire enters the skin. Insert the dilator over the wire and push into the skin as far as it will go. Remove the dilator.
- Insert the central line over the wire. Keep one hand on the wire at all times. When the central line is 2 cm away from the skin, slowly withdraw the wire back through the central line until the wire tip appears from the line port. Hold the wire here while you insert the line. Leave a few centimetres of the line outside the skin. Withdraw the wire and immediately clip off the remaining port.
- Attach the line to the skin with sutures. Tie loosely so as not to pinch the skin; this causes necrosis and detachment of the line. Clean the skin around the line once more, dry and cover with occlusive dressings.
- Ensure that you can aspirate blood from each lumen of the line, then flush each lumen with saline or heparin saline.
- Order a chest X-ray to check for line position and pneumothorax if a jugular or subclavian line has been inserted. Femoral lines do not need X-raying.

Pitfalls

Cannot cannulate the vein: try another site. If you have access to a portable ultrasound device, try using this

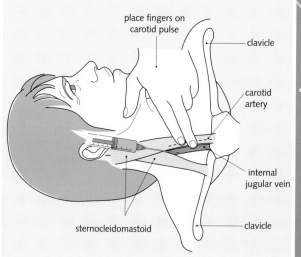

Fig. 31 Placing a central line. Insert the needle lateral to the carotid artery, aiming for the right nipple in men or the anterior superior iliac spine in women. (Adapted from Sprigings D, Chambers J, Jeffrey A. *Acute Medicine*, 2nd edition, 1995 Blackwell Science.)

> Arterial puncture: this is not always obvious, especially in shocked, hypoxic patients, when the blood can be dark and flow sluggishly. If you do hit an artery, remove the needle and press firmly for 5 min with a gauze swab
>
> Vein cannulated but wire fails to advance: sometimes veins are small, tortuous or occluded, e.g. by thrombus from previous cannulation attempts. Do not force the wire; try another site
>
> Line in wrong place: occasionally, lines double back on themselves, or subclavian lines go up into the jugular. If this occurs, either remove the line and start again or, if you have access to fluoroscopic guidance, try and reinsert the wire, remove the line, and reposition the wire
>
> Beware using too much local anaesthetic on multiple line insertions; the maximum dose should not really exceed 3–5 mg/kg; i.e. 10–15 mL of 2% lidocaine for a 70-kg patient

Central lines do not cure patients. They take longer to put in than you think and often require the patient to lie flat with drapes on the head for some time. Make sure that you are treating the patient's condition as well as inserting a central line.

Drug issues

Drug issues

Pain control

A doctor should cure sometimes, relieve often and comfort always. Pain control is therefore a vital part of your job and is often an area where you can make a real difference as a foundation doctor. Pain is complex; different people perceive pain in different ways, and therapy always needs to be individualized. The following are some tips regarding pain control:

- Find out what the cause of the pain is, e.g. metastases, angina, broken rib.
- Don't forget that simple measures are important, e.g. positioning of the patient.
- Anxiety makes pain worse. Listening to people in pain and letting them know that you are there for them is important.
- Regular analgesia to keep pain under control is better than trying to treat pain when it becomes unbearable.

The ladder of analgesia

1. Paracetamol 1 g every 6 h, to a maximum of 4 g every 24 h. This is sufficient for mild pain.
2. Weak opioids, e.g. codeine 30–60 mg every 4–6 h, to a maximum of 180 mg per day.
3. Strong opioids, e.g. morphine. Start with 5 mg every 4 h. Once you have an idea of the daily required dose, change to a long-acting version, e.g. MST every 12 h. Make sure that the doses are equivalent.

Adjunctive therapy

NSAIDs Good for musculoskeletal pain and pleuritic pain, e.g. pericarditis, fracture/sprain, gout. Use the weakest preparation that works for the shortest possible time, e.g. ibuprofen 400 mg three times a day. Avoid if there is GI bleeding, other major bleeding, heart failure, low platelets, iron-deficiency anaemia. Try and avoid in indigestion; you might have to use a gastroprotective agent, e.g. a proton pump inhibitor.

Anxiolytics/sedatives Oral diazepam or, in terminal care, subcutaneous midazolam infusion, are good agents for dealing with severe anxiety that can exacerbate pain.

Don't forget that analgesia, especially opioid analgesia, has side-effects. Give antiemetics and don't start even a weak opioid without giving laxatives at the same time.

If you are having difficulty controlling pain or other bothersome symptoms, call the palliative care team. They are usually very willing to give advice as to suitable analgesic regimens and they always appreciate being involved at an earlier stage, rather than in the hours before someone dies.

Opiate overdose

Overdose of opiates can occur deliberately, as a suicide attempt, or because of rapid increases in dose (as might be seen during the use of a PCA pump, for example). Look for pinpoint pupils, drowsiness and a reduced respiratory rate. Stop the pump if one is in use, and give 400–800 µg of naloxone IV or IM. Naloxone has a relatively short half-life – be prepared to give more as it wears off and, in the case of long-acting morphine preparations, an infusion might be necessary.

Constipation

Constipation is common. Many of your patients will be older and thus likely to suffer from constipation. If they weren't constipated when they came into hospital, they will be after a few days of opioids and bed rest. Keeping people mobile and encouraging them to drink plenty of water (or keeping them otherwise well hydrated) both help to avoid constipation.

There are two traps in constipation. First, is the patient constipated or is there a bowel obstruction? Get an abdominal film if the abdomen is distended or there are other signs of obstruction. Second, constipation can hide – it might not be apparent on PR exam and, in severe cases, overflow diarrhoea can occur. Clearly, in this case, laxatives are needed, rather than medications to try and stem the diarrhoea.

FIRST-LINE AGENTS

Select no more than one from each group; they can be combined.

- Softeners – sodium docusate: 200 mg three times per day.
- Bulking agents – ispaghula husk, e.g. Fybogel: one sachet twice a day; sterculia, e.g. Normacol.
- Stimulants – senna: two tablets at dinnertime; bisacodyl.
- Osmotic laxatives – magnesium hydroxide: 10 mL twice a day; lactulose: 10–20 mL twice a day.

SECOND-LINE AGENTS

- Movicol: contains polyethylene glycol, a water retainer and osmotic laxative.
- Codanthramer, codanthrusate: these combine a softener and danthron, a powerful stimulant. They are sometimes used in patients with terminal disease – danthron carries a theoretical risk of carcinogenicity.
- Glycerin suppository, phosphate enema: good for clearing hard stools from the rectum but insufficient on their own to treat constipation higher up in the bowel.

BOWEL PREPARATION

Your surgical unit or colonoscopy unit will probably have a favourite routine for cleaning the colon. There are two common choices:

- Sodium picosulphate (Picolax): two to three sachets spread over a 24-h period. A potent stimulant, this can cause dehydration, nausea, vomiting, abdominal pain and dizziness. Make sure that your patients are well hydrated; older, frail people might need an IV infusion.
- Polyethylene glycol (e.g. Klean-prep): this is taken with a lot of water (up to 4 L), thus dehydration is less of a problem. Encourage your patients to drink a glassful every 10–15 min; the whole 4 L should be drunk over a 6-h period, which might be difficult for some patients.

Neither of these preparations is designed to combat constipation.

Nausea and vomiting

Before unthinkingly prescribing an antiemetic, ask yourself why the patient is vomiting. Not only will this help you choose an appropriate antiemetic, it might allow you to remove the underlying cause (see 'Nausea and vomiting', p. 166).

(see 'Nausea and vomiting', p. 166)

USEFUL PREPARATIONS

- Metoclopramide 10 mg 8-hourly – oral, subcutaneous, IM or IV: good for most types of nausea and vomiting, including opioid-induced vomiting, gastric stasis (metoclopramide improves gastric emptying), chemotherapy-induced vomiting. Avoid if there is any chance of bowel obstruction or gastric outlet obstruction.

- Prochlorperazine 12.5 mg 12-hourly IM or 5 mg three times a day orally: similar to metoclopramide but without the effects on gastric motility. More useful for vestibular and cerebellar disorders than metoclopramide. Like metoclopramide, it can induce extrapyramidal side-effects and – rarely – dystonic reactions.

- Haloperidol 1–5 mg orally or IM as required: Another alternative to metoclopramide, with a similar mode of action. Useful for intractable nausea, e.g. in cancer patients.

- Granisetron, ondansetron, tropisetron: these drugs all block $5HT_3$ receptors. They are expensive and their use is usually strictly controlled by local policies – check yours. They are useful for chemotherapy- and radiotherapy-induced vomiting, postoperative nausea and vomiting.

- Cyclizine 50 mg three times a day orally, subcutaneously, IM or IV: useful for most types of nausea, including nausea of vestibular or cerebellar origin. Can be sedating, however. Avoid in acute myocardial infarction; may have adverse haemodynamic consequences.

- Hyoscine 200–400 µg twice a day: useful for motion sickness and for reducing secretions into an obstructed gut when surgery cannot be performed.

Anticoagulation

WARFARIN

Warfarin therapy is indicated for treatment of DVT and pulmonary embolism, for reducing the risk of stroke in atrial fibrillation and mural thrombus, to prevent recurrence of other arterial emboli, and to prevent thrombosis of prosthetic heart valves. For most indications, including some more modern prosthetic valves, the target INR is 2–3. Older prosthetic valves and patients with recurrent thrombi due to anticardiolipin syndrome should be maintained at an INR of 3–4:

- Contraindications to warfarin: heavy alcohol intake, increased risk of bleeding (e.g. bladder tumour, known gastric ulcer) and a tendency to fall are relative contraindications to warfarin.

- Taking the INR: the INR should be taken in the morning, as close to 9 a.m. as possible. Dosing nomograms do not work if the sample is taken in the afternoon or evening.

- Dosing time: warfarin should be given at 6 p.m. Make sure that you have prescribed warfarin (usually on a separate prescription chart) before finishing your working day.

- Commencing warfarin: patients should receive an explanation of when to take warfarin, be told about the risks of bleeding, the need for regular blood tests (especially if they change their medications) and be given a record booklet for recording INR and dose. Most warfarin protocols use a loading dose (e.g. 10 mg first day, 10 mg second day), followed by INR testing on days 3, 4 and 5; check your local protocol and beware using high loading doses in older patients. 5 mg per day to load is usually sufficient.

- Blood testing: FBC, INR and LFTs should be performed prior to starting warfarin; patients with liver disease might already be autoanticoagulated. Test daily from day 3 until INR is stable, then two to three times per week, gradually reducing testing to once every 2–4 weeks if stable.

- Drug interactions: many drugs affect warfarin function; drugs such as antibiotics and amiodarone potentiate the effect, whereas carbamazepine reduces the effect of warfarin. Measure the INR frequently whenever changing drugs – both when stopping and starting.

- Warfarin overdose and bleeding: The British Society of Haematology recommends the following approach:
  - INR > 6, no/minor bleeding: stop warfarin and restart when INR < 5
  - INR > 8, no/minor bleeding, but other risk factors for bleeding present: give 0.5–2.5 mg of oral vitamin K. Stop warfarin and restart when INR < 5.
  - Major bleeding: stop warfarin. Give 5 mg vitamin K (IV or oral). Give FFP or prothrombin complex concentrate.

USE OF HEPARIN

- Prophylaxis: consider using prophylactic heparin (5000 U twice daily of unfractionated or a small daily dose of low-molecular-weight heparin) for any patient who is immobile or undergoing significant surgery. Combine with TED stockings.

- Treatment: heparin is used for the acute treatment of venous and arterial thromboembolism (compare this with 'Warfarin', above). It is better to use low-molecular-weight heparin if possible because this gives more reliable dosing and does not require monitoring.

Unfractionated IV heparin is useful when the infusion might need to be switched off quickly, i.e. imminent surgery, high risk of bleeding. Give a bolus dose of 5000 U, then start infusion at 1000 U/h. Take the APTT ratio at 6 h, adjust the dose according to your local protocol. Make sure the APTT ratio is repeated 6 h after every adjustment.

Steroids

Steroids are extremely useful drugs; they are also associated with a wide range of side-effects. Steroid therapy can be divided into short-term and long-term therapy.

Short courses The most common use is for asthma. A 5–10-day course of oral prednisolone, 30–50 mg daily, is typical. Such short courses do not need to be tapered unless the patient is usually on long-term steroids.

Long courses Used for conditions such as temporal arteritis, inflammatory bowel disease and rheumatological diseases. If doses above 7.5 mg per day are administered for longer than a few weeks, suppression of the adrenal axis can occur. Sudden withdrawal in this situation can precipitate an Addisonian crisis. Prevent this from occurring by:

- tapering long-term steroids – do not stop suddenly
- doubling the usual dose of steroid if the patient is admitted unwell or needs surgery
- using IV hydrocortisone 50 mg four times a day if the patient is nil by mouth.

Side-effects of long-term steroids Patients develop a Cushingoid appearance after long-term high-dose steroids. Steroids suppress the immune system, and infections are common in people on long-term steroids. These could involve atypical pathogens and might present insidiously – the normal inflammatory response is damped down.

- Steroids increase blood glucose – check for diabetes with a fasting morning glucose.
- Steroids cause osteoporosis. All patients on long-term steroids (longer than a couple of weeks) should be on a bone-protecting agent (e.g. a bisphosphonate).
- Steroids can increase the WCC; this is not reliable as a guide to infection on its own.

Sedation

Ask yourself why you are prescribing sedatives – is it for the patient, for your convenience, for the nurses' convenience or for the relatives? There are usually good reasons not to prescribe sedatives:

- sedative agents (e.g. benzodiazepines) cause delirium, especially in older patients
- sedatives increase the risk of falls
- sedatives are addictive and can be very difficult to withdraw

When to prescribe sedation

- When the patient is on long-term sedatives for insomnia or anxiety: continue the same prescription (usually a benzodiazepine). If the admission is prolonged, you could consider trying gradually to reduce the dose and wean the patient off the sedative.
- When acute anxiety is causing symptoms: an example would be worsening of chest pains in a patient without coronary artery disease, or anxiety worsening bone pain in metastatic malignancy. Be very careful – it is safer to assume that symptoms cause anxiety, rather than the reverse.
- As premedication before surgery or other invasive procedures: the anaesthetist will often prescribe these, e.g. 5–10 mg diazepam.
- If the patient is agitated and is a danger to him- or herself and to others. Intramuscular agents, e.g. haloperidol 1–3 mg might be necessary.
- If all else has failed and the patient is sleeping badly, an occasional sleeping tablet might be necessary, e.g. temazepam 10 mg or lormetazepam 500 mcg as required.

When not to prescribe sedatives

- Insomnia: this is common in hospital, and sleeping tablets are not always the best answer. Try milky drinks, low lighting, even a tot of whisky before bed.
- Agitated, wandering patient: chemical sedation or restraint often worsens this situation, worsening confusion and precipitating falls. There are also ethical problems with chemical restraint. Treat the cause of the confusion if possible, nurse in familiar surroundings, avoid darkness at night and consider a floor bed to avoid falls.

Special circumstances

- Alcohol withdrawal: use benzodiazepines, and use them early – before withdrawal starts (48–72 h). Diazepam 10–20 mg four times a day, tapering to zero over a 10-day period, is a useful regimen.

Blood and blood products

Ordering and administering blood products should be done with the utmost care and attention. When requesting blood, the forms and specimen bottles should be written correctly, with at least three points of identification on each. Incorrect transfusions unfortunately still occur – do your best to minimize the risk.

Types of blood product

Packed red cells Traditional whole blood is hardly ever used. Packed red cells should be given to those patients who are shocked or otherwise compromised with a low haemoglobin, e.g. trauma, GI bleeds. Patients who are anaemic but are otherwise well do not need a transfusion; they need investigation of their anaemia and appropriate treatment, e.g. iron if iron deficient. If there is an underlying haematological cause for the anaemia, then discuss this with your local haematologist, who will advise appropriately.

- Administration: usually given over 4 h via at least a green (18G) cannula. In patients with heart failure or the elderly, consider giving 20 mg furosemide orally with every other bag.

Platelets Thrombocytopaenia (platelet count of $< 50 \times 10^9$/L) is not an indication for platelet transfusion unless active bleeding is occurring. All patients who are to undergo an invasive procedure in which platelet cover is required should be discussed with your local haematologist. Equally, the underlying reason for the thrombocytopaenia should be sought, e.g. drug reaction (heparin is a common culprit) or marrow suppression.

- Administration: give through at least a pink (20G) cannula over 15–30 min. Usually, 1–2 units are given.

Fresh frozen plasma (FFP) This contains important clotting factors. It is commonly used in patients with liver failure. Use only if a patient is bleeding.

- Administration: give through at least a pink (20G) cannula over 15 min.

Pure factor concentrates: Are usually used now in patients who have become over-anticoagulated with warfarin (e.g. overdose or interaction with antibiotics).

Transfusion reactions

Acute haemolytic transfusion reaction The most serious early transfusion reaction commonly occurs when there is ABO incompatibility, e.g. the wrong patient receiving blood. It manifests itself usually in the first 15 min. The patient will suffer from fever, agitation, flushing, hypotension, breathlessness, abdominal pain and oozing from the cannula site. There is complement activation and DIC.

- Treatment: stop the blood transfusion. Call for senior help; carefully monitor urine output and give IV fluids if urine output is poor. If there is still no urine output, the patient might be developing renal failure and will need CVP monitoring. Perform an ECG, check K^+ and treat with insulin and dextrose if hyperkalaemic.

Non-haemolytic febrile transfusion reactions Fever and rigors occur in about 1–2% of transfusions. This is usually a result of immunity to white cells developed during previous transfusions or in pregnancy.

- Treatment: slow or stop the blood and give paracetamol.

Allergic reactions

Generalized allergic reactions, e.g. urticaria, occur just as in other drug administrations.

- Treatment: stop the blood and give 10 mg IV chlorpheniramine $\pm$ 100 mg IV hydrocortisone.

Fluid overload

Patients with heart failure and the elderly should be transfused with caution. If there is fluid overload, e.g. pulmonary oedema, treat with IV furosemide.

Late complications

These are not common and include iron overload and antibody development (in patients with repeated transfusions), graft versus host disease and infections.

Infections, although uncommon, are often a patient's greatest fear about a transfusion. Reassure the patient that all blood is now screened for all major infections, e.g. HIV and hepatitis B. You should, however, bear in mind that transfusions should be used only when absolutely necessary – there might well be undiscovered blood-borne infections.

Medical emergencies

Medical emergencies

Cardiac arrest

Being prepared is key – familiarize yourself with the defibrillators in your Trust. The older monophasic defibrillators have hand-held paddles and use the traditional 200J and 360J energy settings for shock delivery. The more modern biphasic defibrillators are safer with pads and lower energy requirements though these settings can vary depending on the maufacturer's recommendations. If there is any doubt, use the energy values given below.

The arrest situation itself is almost always chaotic, with people rushing about and no apparent order to things. You will probably be the first doctor there.

Organize your thoughts and then organize the arrest; the rest of your team will not be far behind.

Diagnosis

Check that the patient has actually arrested – check the pulse and confirm that the patient is not breathing.

What to do

- If you witness the arrest, give a precordial thump. If the arrest is unwitnessed, start chest compressions and use a bag-and-mask to ventilate (30 compressions to 2 ventilations). Ask for the cardiac monitor and check the rhythm. Decide if the rhythm is VT/VF or something else (PEA – Pulseless Electrical Activity):
  - VT/VF:
    - Place pads/paddles on chest and give a single shock (360J).
    - Recommence CPR immediately (30:2) and continue for 2 min.
    - If VT/VF persists, give a second shock (360J). Check the pulse only if there is a change in the rhythm. Resume CPR for 2 min.
    - If VT/VF persists give 1 mg Adrenaline (10 mL of 1:10 000) and give 3rd shock (360J). Recheck monitor. If still VT/VF continue CPR for 2 min.
    - If VT/VF persists, give Amiodarone 300 mg IV followed by 4th shock. Continue CPR for 2 min if VF/VT persists.
  - PEA:
    - Get venous access. Give 1 mg adrenaline IV (10 mL of 1:10 000) immediately.
    - Is the patient in asystole or PEA with a heart rate < 60 bpm? If so give 3 mg Atropine IV
    - Continue CPR (30:2) until airway is secure then perform continuous compressions without pausing during ventilation

This should get you through the first few frantic minutes. Step back and think about what is going on:

If the patient remains in VT/VF despite 4 shocks and amiodarone:

- Continue 2-min cycles of CPR with 360J shocks in between cycles if VT/VF persists
- Give 1 mg Adrenaline IV with every other shock
- Find out the last K^+ and Mg^{2+} results and correct if necessary.

If the patient changes rhythm to some form of organized electrical activity – check pulse.

- A patient who remains pulseless in any rhythm other than VT/VF remains in PEA. You have more time:

    - Continue 2-min cycles of CPR with 1 mg Adrenaline with every other cycle.

Think about the correctable factors to have caused PEA:

- Get a history: chances are you don't know the patient. Tell someone to get you the notes. Make sure they belong to the patient who has arrested.
- Go through the correctible factors in turn:

THE FOUR 'Hs'

- Hypoxia: the patient is already being ventilated but might need intubation.
- Hypovolaemia: run the fluids in quickly. Use a large peripheral cannula in a big vein. Is the patient bleeding? If so, where from?
- Hyperkalaemia, hypocalcaemia, acidaemia: get the latest set of U+Es and send off blood gases
- Hypothermia

THE FOUR 'Ts'

- Tension pneumothorax: listen for reduced air movement on one side and feel for tracheal deviation
- Cardiac tamponade
- Toxic substances or therapeutic substances in overdose
- Thromboembolic (e.g. pulmonary embolus)

COMMON CAUSES OF IN-HOSPITAL CARDIAC ARRESTS OUTSIDE THE CCU

- Pulmonary embolism
- Pump failure/cardiac rupture from myocardial infarction
- Bleeding

Points to watch

No venous access Try a venflon in the femoral vein or external jugular vein – it is often distended. Give drugs down the endotracheal tube.
Unclear whether rhythm is asystole or fine VF Push the gain right up on the monitor and reassess. If there is still doubt, do NOT shock the patient. Continue CPR (30:2).
P-waves on monitor but no QRS complex and no output Put on temporary pacing pads for external pacing. Increase the threshold until you get QRS complexes – this usually results in the chest muscles twitching. Call for senior help; this patient needs a temporary pacing wire.

Successful resuscitation

You regain a cardiac output. Look at the patient:

- Is the patient beginning to breathe unaided? If not, the patient will need ITU.
- Is the patient waking up?
- Measure the blood pressure.

- Get a 12-lead ECG and look for an underlying MI. Consider thrombolysis unless the arrest is very prolonged.
- Send off a blood gas and get a chest X-ray; discuss further management with your registrar.

Failed resuscitation

Your senior should be present to make the decision to stop resuscitating. You should continue, particularly if there is a shockable rhythm. The decision to stop should be made with all of the team managing the arrest. You need to make sure that the patient's relatives have been contacted. You should take notes and document the arrest – this will give time for nurses to clean the patient and prepare for family. Record the:

- time the call was put out
- circumstances in which the patient was found – witnessed or not; if not, when the patient was last seen
- initial rhythm
- nature and results of treatment given
- time the resuscitation attempt was abandoned.

Go back to the patient and certify death. Document the time of death.

TALKING TO THE RELATIVES

- Leave your bleep with someone. Introduce yourself and explain the circumstances of the arrest and management. Don't use technical language. Be compassionate; they do not need gory details.
- Be prepared to take some time. You might not be able to answer all of their questions, particularly if it is not your patient.

Arrests are traumatic events for everyone. Don't worry about showing emotion; someone has died and it is perfectly normal to be emotional in these circumstances.

Acute MI

Assess all patients with chest pain immediately, even if only to check their vital signs and ECG. 'Time is myocardium'.

Diagnosis

The diagnosis is made on the history and ECG. Cardiac enzymes (CK, CK-MB and troponins) are unhelpful in deciding whether to thrombolyse; they are a retrospective guide to diagnosis. ECG criteria for thrombolysis are:

- ≥ 2 mm ST elevation in two or more of the chest leads (V_1–V_6)
- ≥ 1 mm ST elevation in two or more of limb leads (II, III and aVF or I and aVL)
- New left bundle branch block.

What to do

- Take a brief history: type of pain, time of onset, previous episodes of pain, contraindications for thrombolysis, previous thrombolysis, allergies.
- Examine the patient quickly but include the vital signs (including both arm blood pressures), JVP, heart and lung examinations, all peripheral pulses and O_2 saturations. If the diagnosis is clear, your plan should be:
  - cardiac monitor
  - 100% O_2 via reservoir mask (caution if COPD)
  - IV access and send bloods for FBC, clotting, U+Es, glucose, lipids. Do a capillary blood glucose (BM). Check a serum troponin 12 hours after pain onset.
  - 2.5–5 mg IV diamorphine or 5–10 mg IV morphine with 10 mg IV metoclopromide for pain
  - 300 mg aspirin PO stat followed by 75 mg od therafter
  - 300 mg clopidogrel PO stat followed by 75 mg od for 1 month
  - organize a portable chest X-ray.
- Ensure there are no contraindications for thrombolysis:
  - active bleeding, e.g. trauma, melaena
  - suspected aortic dissection
  - prolonged resuscitation
  - recent head trauma or suspicion of intracranial haemorrhage
  - pregnancy
  - blood pressure > 200/120; give IV nitrates to reduce blood pressure, then thrombolyse
  - recent major trauma or surgery (e.g. laparotomy within 2 weeks)
  - recent stroke (within 6–8 weeks or previous haemorrhagic stroke)
  - active proliferative diabetic retinopathy – discuss with your seniors.
- If no contraindications give thrombolysis. Most hospital use a bolus throbolytic based on tissue plasminogen activator (tPA). Some may still use streptokinase (SK) 1.5 MU. Check your local guidelines.

If BM > 10, then start an insulin sliding scale even if there is no history of diabetes. Move the patient to the CCU.

Points to watch post-thrombolysis

Hypotension This is common with streptokinase. Stop the infusion and, if the blood pressure improves, restart at half the rate. If the blood pressure remains low, consider giving tPA. Haemorrhage is an alternative cause of hypotension.

Allergic reaction Stop thrombolysis. Give IV chlorpheniramine 10 mg and IV hydrocortisone 100 mg.

Reduced GCS This strongly suggests intracranial bleeding – stop thrombolysis and call your senior; an urgent CT head is needed.

Bleeding Into the gut, urinary tract or from vascular puncture. Stop infusion and give blood and FFP/aprotinin. Get advice from your local haematologist.

Points to watch post-MI

HYPOTENSION

This might be due to bleeding or to primary cardiogenic shock.

- Give IV colloid via a large peripheral cannula in case of obvious bleeding.
- Call for senior advice if no obvious bleeding seen. Get an urgent echo to assess the LV function.
- Repeat 12-lead ECG.
- Put in urinary catheter to measure urine hourly.
- The patient might need a central line or Swan–Ganz catheter plus inotropic support.

PULMONARY OEDEMA

- Give furosemide (frusemide) IV 80 mg. Call senior help.
- Listen for new systolic murmurs of VSD or acute mitral regurgitation. Get an urgent echo.
- If not improving, give another 80 mg furosemide (frusemide) IV and start an IV nitrate infusion (50 mg GTN in 50 mL N Saline infused at 2–10 mg/h).

RIGHT VENTRICULAR INFARCTION

Low blood pressure with raised JVP, but the chest is often clear. Do a right-sided ECG and look for ST elevation in V_4R; this indicates RV infarction. Give IV fluids, not diuretics in this situation. Try 250 mL of colloid over 15 min.

RHYTHM DISTURBANCES

Symptomatic bradycardia Give IV atropine 0.5 mg every 5 min to a maximum of 3 mg total. If still bradycardic, proceed to temporary pacing.

Complete heart block In anterior MI or if symptomatic or haemodynamically compromised, put in a temporary pacing wire; otherwise observe on the CCU.

Ventricular tachycardia Call for senior help. If asymptomatic, give IV amiodarone. If symptomatic, the patient needs immediate cardioversion. Note that accelerated idioventricular rhythm ('slow VT') at around 90–120 per min is common in the hours after an MI and does not usually require treatment.

CHEST PAIN

Pericarditis ECG shows saddling of ST segments. The pain is sharp and worse on leaning forward, lying flat, and on inspiration. Give NSAIDs, e.g. diclofenac 50 mg three times a day.

Angina ECG shows no resolution of ST segments, or re-elevation of ST segments. Call for senior review – the patient might need rethrombolysing or urgent angioplasty.

Musculoskeletal Point tenderness on chest – treat with simple analgesia.

Acute coronary syndromes

Acute coronary syndromes include a spectrum of patients presenting with cardiac chest pain. Included within this group are patients with typical chest pain with no diagnostic ECG changes, patients with chest pain with serum troponin elevation and ST segment depression on their ECGs, and non-Q-wave MIs.

Diagnosis

The diagnosis is made on the history. The ECG might be normal on presentation. Initial assessment should include a review of the ECG together with a review of vital signs.

What to do

- Take a brief history including some specific questions:
  - is the patient known to have ischaemic heart disease? If so, is the pain like normal angina?
  - if not, has the patient had this pain before? Has the patient been investigated for this pain? If so, what tests?
  - how long has the patient had the pain? Has it become more frequent recently? Has the patient had the pain at rest?
  - does rest or GTN make the pain go away?
- Summarize the patient's risk factors. What tablets is the patient taking? Has the patient stopped taking them for any reason?
- Examine the patient's cardiovascular and respiratory systems carefully. Look particularly for signs of aortic stenosis and anaemia (non-coronary artery disease causes of angina). Check blood pressure in both arms and all peripheral pulses looking for signs of aortic dissection. Look for other causes of chest pain (e.g. COPD and pneumonia).
- Insert cannula and send bloods for FBC, U+Es, lipids, clotting. Send a serum troponin 12 hours after pain onset.
- Look at the ECG – specifically for ST depression. Unstable angina can also show non-specific T-wave inversion, which might be significant, especially if it is reversible.
- Chest X-ray – look for a widened mediastinum in case of aortic dissection. Check the apices for a small pneumothorax. Look for signs of pneumonia.
- Do arterial blood gases if O_2 saturations are low (< 95%) or the history suggests a primary lung diagnosis, e.g. pulmonary embolism, pneumonia, COPD, or pulmonary oedema.

Management

- Put the patient on a cardiac monitor. Give 100% O_2, IV diamorphine 2.5–5 mg plus IV metoclopramide 10 mg and aspirin 300 mg PO stat followed by 75 mg once daily thereafter. Get a chest X-ray if this has not been done.

- Give either low-molecular-weight heparin (enoxaparin or tinzaparin) or unfractionated heparin 5000 U as bolus followed by 24 000 U over 24 h. The APTT ratio must be checked every 6 h and be between 1.5 and 2.5 if you are using unfractionated heparin.
- If the patient is still complaining of pain, start IV nitrates 50 mg in 50 mL of normal saline infused at 2–10 mg/h. Titrate to pain and blood pressure, aiming to keep systolic BP > 100 mmHg.
- If the patient has ST depression on ECG, give clopidogrel 300 mg stat followed by 75 mg once daily.
- Keep on cardiac monitor if troponin is elevated.
- Commence sliding scale of insulin if the capillary blood glucose > 10.
- If not already on a beta-blocker, and there is no history of asthma, COPD or heart failure, start a small dose (e.g. atenolol 25 mg once daily).

FURTHER MANAGEMENT

- Do a troponin at 12 h post-onset of chest pain, together with a repeat ECG. Exact timing can vary; see your local hospital policy.
- Do an ECG the following morning and daily as long as the patient remains an inpatient.

Points to watch

- Look for poor prognostic features such as:
  - hypotension when in pain
  - reversible ST segment elevation with pain
  - pain despite high doses of IV nitrates.
- If the patient has dynamic ECG changes, i.e. ST elevation when in pain and/or a drop in blood pressure, then call for senior help. This patient might need treatment with a GPIIb/IIIa antagonist and discussion with a specialist cardiology centre for consideration for urgent angiography.
- If the patient is tachycardic (pulse > 90 per min) then consider giving IV beta-blockers, e.g. metoprolol 12.5 mg IV and 25 mg three times a day thereafter. Avoid if there is a history of COPD, asthma or heart failure.

Acute left ventricular failure

Diagnosis

Patients presenting with LVF often present in the early hours of the morning. Correct initial assessment is crucial and response to treatment is often dramatic. Look for basal crackles, a raised JVP and cool peripheries.

What to do

- Assess the patient's airway and vital signs. Call for senior help if the patient is hypotensive (systolic BP < 90 mmHg). If SaO_2 < 90% then perform ABGs. If pO_2 < 8 kPa, pH < 7.3 or pCO_2 > 6 then call for senior help.

- Examine the patient rapidly, looking for signs of pulmonary oedema. Exclude any other diagnosis, e.g. exacerbation of COPD, pneumonia. Note that it is not uncommon for patients with pulmonary oedema to have wheeze, and inspiratory crackles might not be heard. This can lead to a mistaken diagnosis of asthma/COPD. Check the chest X-ray if you are unsure.

- Put the patient on a cardiac monitor. Give 60–80% O_2 via non-rebreathing (reservoir) bag and maintain saturations > 95% or pO_2 > 8 kPa. Be cautious in patients with COPD.

- Perform a 12-lead ECG – look for any evidence of myocardial infarction or arrhythmia. Send urgent bloods for FBC, U+Es, glucose, Mg^{2+}, and 12 hour troponin.

- Get an urgent chest X-ray – look for signs of pulmonary oedema, e.g. upper lobe diversion, bilateral lung shadowing and blunting of costophrenic angles. Exclude other diagnoses, such as pneumothorax and pneumonia. Pleural effusions need to be tapped to identify their cause.

- If the patient is unwell, chest X-ray confirmation of pulmonary oedema is not necessary. Treat the patient on clinical grounds.

- Give diamorphine 2.5–5 mg IV, metoclopramide 10 mg IV, furosemide (frusemide) 80 mg IV. Repeat after 30 min if necessary. If systolic BP >100 mmHg and pulmonary oedema is not settling, start a GTN infusion (50 mg GTN in 50 mL normal saline at 2–10 mg/min IV). Monitor BP closely.

- If an MI or arrhythmia is seen on the ECG, this should be treated quickly. Heparin (unfractionated or LMWH) should be considered if there is a history of chest pain, even if the ECG is normal.

- Patients with a systolic blood pressure < 90 mmHg are in cardiogenic shock. Call for senior help immediately. The patient will need a central line and you should insert a urinary catheter to monitor the patient's urine output. Consider inotropic support with dobutamine 5 µg/kg/min increasing slowly every 2–3 min by 2.5 µg/kg/min to a maximum of 20 µg/kg/min. Echocardiography should be performed to look at LV function and to exclude a pericardial effusion.

- If the patient does not respond to initial therapy, or is in respiratory failure with a low pH and rising pCO_2 on arterial blood gases, non-invasive positive pressure ventilation is required. Talk to your seniors urgently; it is better to start this sooner rather than later.

Some causes of pulmonary oedema:

• Myocardial infarction or severe ischaemia • Arrhythmia with or without underlying LV dysfunction • Acute valve lesions, e.g. aortic regurgitation due to aortic dissection or endocarditis, mitral regurgitation due to chordae rupture • Ventricular septal defect rupture post-MI • Severe aortic stenosis • Poor compliance with drug therapy • Excess IV fluid administration, e.g. perioperatively • 'Flash' pulmonary oedema from renal artery stenosis • Oliguric renal failure

Once the initial attack has been treated, the cause for the acute episode should be found. Do serial ECGs to exclude any evidence of ischaemia or infarction, along with troponin measurements at presentation and 6–12 h later if the first test is normal. Get an echocardiogram to look at LV function and valves and to check for any deterioration if a pre-existing condition is present. If LV function is normal, get a 24 h Holter monitor to exclude arrhythmias.

Arrhythmias

There are two broad categories of arrhythmias: bradyarrhythmias and tachyarrhythmias. Arrhythmia management can be complicated and there are plenty of cardiologists who argue amongst themselves in this regard. The following are some basic rules to be applied in their diagnosis and management.

Diagnosis of tachyarrhythmias

The heart rate is fast: > 120 bpm. Make sure that there are no P waves on the ECG (i.e. that it is not a sinus tachycardia).

WHAT TO DO

In all of these patients, a full drug history should be taken, including recreational drug use. A 12-lead ECG should be performed and the diagnosis made. Urgent blood tests, including U+Es, Mg^{2+}, 12-hour troponin, should be sent.

- If the patient is compromised (systolic BP < 90 mmHg, pulmonary oedema or chest pain): call for senior help immediately – the patient is periarrest and should undergo DC cardioversion.

- If the patient is not compromised: identification of the rhythm is important for diagnosis and treatment of tachyarrhythmias. There are certain questions you should ask yourself:
  - look at the QRS complex: is it narrow or broad? Narrow complex tachycardias are SVTs. AF is a type of SVT and is irregular in its rate. The remainder are regular in nature. If the rate is ≈ 150 per min and regular, the diagnosis is highly likely to be atrial flutter with 2:1 block.

MANAGEMENT OF ATRIAL FIBRILLATION VENTRICULAR RATE > 120 bpm

- Give the patient adequate O_2 and put onto a cardiac monitor.
- Load with digoxin: 500 µg stat PO (250 µg if elderly or in renal failure); 250 µg at 6 h; 250 µg at 12 h; 125 µg regular daily dose.
- Alternatives include beta-blockers, diltiazem and amiodarone.

MANAGEMENT OF SVT AND ATRIAL FLUTTER

- Give the patient O_2 to maintain adequate oxygenation. Put onto a cardiac monitor.
- If there are no contraindications, e.g. asthma/COPD, give adenosine 3 mg as a rapid IV bolus while recording the patient's rhythm. If there is no change, give 6 mg, then 9 mg, then 12 mg. Adenosine will either cardiovert the rhythm or slow the rate down to demonstrate flutter waves. Warn the patient it might cause transient chest pain and a sense of feeling unwell for a few seconds.
- If cardioversion does not occur and there are no demonstrable flutter waves, you will have to call your seniors to consider alternatives, e.g. verapamil or beta-blockers.

BROAD COMPLEX TACHYCARDIA

Broad complex tachycardia is a little more difficult. The differential diagnosis is:

- Ventricular tachycardia (VT).
- SVT with aberrant conduction, e.g. pre-existing or rate-related bundle branch block.

Features suggesting VT:

- Recent MI ● Previous history of IHD or VT ● ECG changes suggestive of VT
- Fusion beats ● Capture beats ● Lead concordance ● Extreme axis deviation

---

- If you are in any doubt at all, treat as VT. Broad complex tachycardias are VT in 90% of cases and the treatment for VT will often work for SVTs as well.
- If the patient is compromised, call your senior urgently and prepare for urgent DC cardioversion. If the patient is not compromised:
  - give O_2 and maintain adequate oxygenation. Put on a cardiac monitor and call your senior
  - give amiodarone IV as bolus then continuous infusion. The patient will usually require a central line for large venous access. Give 300 mg in 5% dextrose over 1 h, then 900 mg in 1 L 5% dextrose over 23 h
  - if the patient is still in VT, alternatives such as beta-blockers or DC cardioversion should be considered.

Diagnosis of bradyarrhythmias

The heart rate is slow: < 60 bpm.

WHAT TO DO

If the patient is unwell (systolic BP < 90 mmHg, low urine output (< 30 mL/h) or reduced level of consciousness):

- Give atropine 500 µg IV. Repeat with 500 µg IV at 5-min intervals to a maximum of 3 mg. If there is no response, the patient requires temporary pacing. If the patient is compromised, you will need to pace with external pacers on the defibrillator.
- Think of the cause. Is it related to a recent MI, particularly an inferior MI? What drugs is the patient taking, e.g. digoxin, diltiazem, verapamil, beta-blockers (including eye-drops; see 'Bradycardias', p. 164). Has the patient taken an overdose? Is the patient hypothyroid? Is there any electrolyte abnormality?

Do not rush into treatment if the patient is not compromised; asymptomatic brady-cardia does not need treating. The causes (see above) should be investigated and, depending on the rhythm, should be discussed further for a permanent pacemaker.

Diabetic ketoacidosis (DKA)

Think of DKA in any person with type 1 diabetes who is unwell. Also consider DKA in patients who are breathless but not hypoxic.

Diagnosis

1. Raised blood glucose (you must send a lab sample; capillary blood glucose readings can be falsely low in DKA).
2. Ketones (ideally in the blood, but urine will do).
3. Metabolic acidosis (pH < 7.30 or bicarbonate < 22) on blood gases.

If all three of the above are present, the patient has DKA. If one is missing, the diagnosis is not DKA.

What to do

- Quick assessment of the patient: pulse, BP, respiratory rate, conscious level, temperature. If the patient is comatose and the respiratory rate is slowing, put out a crash call – the patient is about to arrest.
- Check the airway and administer high-flow O_2. Put in at least one large bore cannula. Take bloods for U+Es, FBC, glucose and blood cultures. Check an ECG.
- Give 1 L of 0.9% saline as fast as possible. As this is running, set up a sliding insulin scale. Local protocols vary but starting an insulin infusion at 6 units/h is a good start. By the time the first litre of saline has run in, the potassium result should be available. A suggested fluid and potassium regimen is:
  - 1 L normal saline: stat
  - 1 L normal saline: over 1 h
  - 1 L normal saline: over 2 h
  - 1 L normal saline: over 4 h
  - 1 L normal saline: over 6 h
- Add potassium as follows:
  - K^+ < 3.0: 40 mmol per bag
  - K^+ 3.0–4.0: 30 mmol per bag
  - K^+ 4.0–5.0: 20 mmol per bag
  - K^+ > 5.0: none

Other aspects of management

- Check blood gases/venous bicarbonate, potassium and glucose at 1 h and every 1–2 h for the first few hours – potassium levels might fall rapidly once insulin is commenced. Do not rely on potassium measurements from the blood gas machine. Warn the lab that the sample is on its way.
- Monitor the patient in a high-dependency environment – cardiac monitor and urinary catheter are essential. The patient might become tired after a few hours of acidotic breathing – close observation is required to detect this. Tiring patients can deteriorate rapidly and might require intubation.

- Do an hourly pulse, BP and urine output. A urinary catheter should be used if the patient is tachycardic, hypotensive, drowsy or fails to pass urine in the first couple of hours.
- Consider a CVP line if the systolic blood pressure is < 90, blood results suggest acute renal failure or urine output fails to pick up after a few hours.
- Do not give bicarbonate without discussing with your seniors first – fluids and insulin are the best way to correct the acidosis. If it must be given then it is usually in patients with a pH < 7.0 (500 mL 1.26% bicarbonate solution with 20 mmol KCl over 30 min IV to a maximum of 2 L) with repeat blood gases.
- Look for a precipitating cause, e.g. infection, MI. Get urine culture, blood cultures and a chest X-ray, inspect the feet and treat any infection. Perform an ECG. Nasogastric tubes are not usually needed but a few patients will have gastric stasis and vomiting, and a tube might 'decompress' the stomach.
- If blood glucose drops to less than 11, switch to IV dextrose but continue the insulin infusion. You will need to reduce the rate to 2–3 units per hour.
- Most hospitals have a protocol for managing DKA; follow it, and involve your seniors early.

Points to watch

- Most problems occur because fluids and insulin are not administered in good time. Get the IV access and the first bag of fluid going while you do blood gases and send bloods off.
- DKA causes a raised WCC; this is not a reliable marker of infection.
- Amylase can rise in DKA, and DKA can cause abdominal pain. Beware making a diagnosis of acute pancreatitis unless the amylase level is very high.
- Some patients exhibit a rapid fall in glucose levels but remain acidotic and ketotic. They require continuing high levels of insulin to switch off ketone production; give 10% dextrose and 6–8 U/h of insulin.
- Serum sodium often rises in DKA. Do not change to 0.45% saline unless serum sodium is above 155 mmol/L.
- Fluid shifts caused by overly aggressive rehydration can lead to cerebral oedema on rare occasions; this might be more common in children and adolescents. Be alert for headache or worsening drowsiness, especially if other biochemical indices are improving.
- Beware older patients with high sugars and few ketones – they often have HONK, not DKA (see below). Also beware older patients on metformin, who might be acidotic with few or no ketones. They might have lactic acidosis – measure the lactate (discuss with the laboratory before sending the sample).

Hyperosmolar non-ketotic state (HONK)

Think of this in any type 2 diabetic who is unwell.

Diagnosis

- Raised blood glucose (on laboratory sample).
- Not acidotic on blood gases.
- Absence of large amount of ketones in urine.
- Raised osmolality (don't request a measured osmolality). Osmolality = 2 (Na + K) + urea + glucose. Normal = 285–295 mOsm/L

What to do

- Quickly take a history and examine the patient. Check pulse, BP, and look carefully for a precipitating cause.

Common precipitants of HONK

- Myocardial infarction • Pneumonia • UTI • Cellulitis • Gastroenteritis • Stroke • Non-adherence to oral hypoglycaemics

- Set up an IV line and take bloods for FBC, U+Es, glucose, CRP. Pass a urinary catheter, perform an ECG and order a chest X-ray. Take blood and urine for culture if pyrexial.
- There is less hurry to rehydrate patients with HONK but they are often more dehydrated than patients with DKA (often 9–10 L deficit). They usually have a very high sodium; beware of bringing this down too quickly. Aim to replace the fluid deficit over 48 h; 1 L of normal saline every 4 h is a good starting point. Avoid dextrose; the sodium might fall too quickly.
- Set up an IV insulin (e.g. Actrapid) infusion, running at 3 units/h. Patients with HONK are much more sensitive to insulin than patients with DKA.
- Check sodium, potassium and glucose after 1 h, then every 2–4 h.
- Give a full dose (not a prophylactic dose) of low-molecular-weight heparin. Patients with HONK are at very high risk of thromboembolism.
- Treat any infection aggressively.

Points to watch

- Consider CVP monitoring if the systolic blood pressure is < 90 mmHg, urine output does not improve after 2–3 L of fluid or if U+Es suggest acute renal failure.
- Consider switching to 0.45% NaCl if the sodium level is > 155 and is not falling with normal saline.
- HONK has a 60% mortality rate, often due to the precipitating condition. Paint a realistic picture to the relatives.
- Blood glucose can fall very quickly once insulin is started; you might need to adjust the insulin infusion rate downwards.

Status epilepticus

Diagnosis

The diagnosis is a clinical one. Do not assume that prolonged generalized epileptiform seizures are pseudoseizures; always treat as status epilepticus.

What to do

- Ensure that the patient cannot be hurt during the seizure; remove nearby obstacles.
- Give 100% O_2. Check the blood glucose (BM stick). If you cannot do this, administer 50 mL of 50% dextrose IV.
- Try and obtain IV access; you will almost certainly need help with this.
- Administer 5 mg of IV diazepam. If seizure activity continues after 2–3 min, administer another 5 mg of diazepam.
- If you cannot obtain IV access quickly, give 5–10 mg of diazepam rectally as a suppository.
- If seizure activity continues, administer fosphenytoin (15 mg of phenytoin equivalent/kg at 150 mg/min) or IV phenytoin 15 mg/kg up to a maximum of 1 g over 20 min.
- If seizure activity continues, you will need expert help. Call an anaesthetist, who might need to paralyse and intubate while giving an anaesthetic such as thiopentone. Try and contact a neurologist; further antiepileptic drugs might be needed and, once anaesthetized, EEG monitoring is often needed to ascertain whether seizure activity is ongoing.

WHEN THE FIT HAS STOPPED

- Check the airway is patent and insert a Guedel airway if not. The patient will almost certainly have a low GCS postictally. Check pulse, BP and O_2 saturations. Take blood for U+Es, FBC, glucose, calcium and blood gases. If you are unsure whether an attack is a pseudoseizure, ask for a prolactin level; this is transiently raised after a genuine seizure in some but not all fits.
- Examine the patient and obtain a collateral history. Bilateral upgoing plantars and a low GCS are normal. Lateralizing signs (e.g. unilateral dilated pupil) suggest an intracranial mass lesion or bleed – get an urgent CT scan of the brain.
- Start a slow IV infusion to keep the line open.

Points to watch

- Clonic activity might die away after a while as the muscles become fatigued – look at the eyelids to see if a fine tremor persists.
- CK and WCC are often raised after a fit; a pyrexia of up to 38°C is also common.

Meningococcal sepsis/meningitis

Diagnosis

Patients with meningococcal sepsis can present with:

- meningitis
- rash and severe sepsis
- both of the above together.

A purpuric rash in an unwell patient is meningococcus. You must administer antibiotics within minutes.

Meningococcaemia – what to do

- Start with ABC (see Chapter 'Medical presentations', p. 152 for a full explanation). The patient might have a compromised airway if their GCS is low. Breathing might be shallow and rapid due to metabolic acidosis. Blood pressure could be low; tachycardia is common. Peripheries can be cool or warm.

- Put in a large bore cannula, take blood cultures and bloods for FBC, clotting (check for DIC), U+Es, CK, LFTs, glucose and CRP. Take an extra FBC tube for meningococcal PCR testing. Start a fast bag of IV saline running; run a bag of colloid in as quickly as possible if the systolic BP is < 90.

- Take a brief history of the condition, past medical history and drug history. Give antibiotics as soon as possible. Cefotaxime 2 g IV is a reasonable choice; consult your local protocol.

- Examine the neurological and abdominal systems. Meningococcal disease can produce abdominal tenderness. Check for GCS, plantars, pupil responses, neck stiffness, photophobia and Kernig's sign.

- Nurse the patient in a high-dependency area; tell your senior as soon as possible – it is a good idea to let ITU know that patients with meningococcal sepsis are around, as they can deteriorate with frightening speed.

- Patients with suspected meningococcal disease should be barrier nursed until they have received > 24 h of IV antibiotics.

- There is no need to proceed to lumbar puncture if the patient has a purpuric rash – the diagnosis is fairly certain and time is of the essence in commencing treatment. Remember that a negative lumbar puncture does not exclude meningococcal disease.

Points to watch

Take an arterial blood gas; metabolic acidosis is common. Insert a urinary catheter if BP < 90, creatinine is raised, or patient has not passed urine within the first 12 h. Insert a central line if the systolic BP < 90 and does not respond to 1 L of colloid. By this point, you should have called your senior, who should be on the phone to the ITU.

Meningitis – what to do

- If the patient has signs of meningism (neck stiffness, positive Kernig's sign, photophobia and headache), start with ABC.

- Does the patient have a rash? If the rash is purpuric, assume that you are dealing with meningococcal disease and proceed as above.

- Otherwise, take a history – was there a prodromal illness, any contacts with meningitis. Any history of foreign travel or head injury? Did the headache come on over hours, or instantly? (see 'Headache', p. 189 for some other useful pointers).

- Examine the patient – abdomen and a full neurological examination. Are there any lateralizing neurological signs to suggest intracranial bleeding or encephalitis. What is the temperature?

- Insert a cannula, take blood cultures, FBC, clotting, U+Es, CRP, glucose, LFTs and an extra FBC tube for meningococcal PCR testing.

- If the patient has a history compatible with intracranial bleeding or a reduced GCS or lateralizing neurological signs, then a CT scan of the brain is required before the lumbar puncture. If the CT scan is clear, or none of the above features are present, carry out a lumbar puncture. Make sure that you phone the request to the duty microbiology technician and ask to be bleeped with the results of microscopy.

- If there is any significant delay in performing the lumbar puncture (i.e. > 30 min between seeing the patient and doing the lumbar puncture), *or* the patient is unwell, give IV antibiotics. Check your local protocol or, if in doubt, give 2 g of IV cefotaxime. Do not wait for the CT, ward round, nursing handover, etc. If necessary, get on and give the antibiotics yourself.

- Patients with a reduced GCS and meningitis should be discussed early with an expert (infection physician or neurologist). Steroids or mannitol might be required.

- If you suspect that someone is immunocompromised (e.g. leukaemia, lymphoma, chemotherapy, HIV), call for expert help early. The differential is wider, and includes *Listeria*, aseptic meningitis, TB, *Cryptococcus* and other fungal infections.

Points to watch

- Meningitis is painful. Give codeine-based analgesia together with paracetamol, e.g. cocodamol 30/500 mg every 6 h.

- Fitting might occur. Treat as per usual with diazepam, and phenytoin if seizures keep occurring. Consider other contributory causes – hypoglycaemia, low sodium, alcohol withdrawal. Consider whether this could be encephalitis – discuss with your seniors.

- Rehydrate the patient, but take care not to overhydrate.

Liver failure

Diagnosis

Suspect this in anyone who is unwell with a previous history of liver disease, or anyone who is confused with abnormal clotting or LFTs. LFTs might be normal in liver failure. Involve a gastroenterologist early; liver failure is complicated to manage, might require ITU involvement, and could need transplantation.

What to do

- Start with ABC. If the patient is unconscious, see 'The unconscious patient', p. 170.
- Take a brief history; speak to a relative if the patient is confused or comatose. Ask about alcohol use, recent bingeing, previous liver disease, any overdoses or changes in medication. Also ask about any family history of liver disease, ingestion of wild mushrooms or herbal medicines, exposure to dry-cleaning fluid. Has the patient been hypotensive recently, or had an anaesthetic?
- Examine the patient: pulse, BP, chest examination for infection, O_2 saturations. Feel for hepatomegaly, splenomegaly, ascites. Do a PR. Is asterixis present? What is the GCS? If normal, carry out a test of higher brain function (e.g. copy a five-pointed star). Are there any focal neurological signs? Patients with liver disease are prone to intracerebral bleeding. Look for evidence of head injury.
- Gain IV access. Send bloods for FBC, INR, LFTs, albumin, calcium, glucose, magnesium, phosphate, group and save. Take blood cultures if pyrexial.
- Do a capillary blood glucose reading and recheck 1–2-hourly. Measure arterial blood gases.
- If the cause of liver failure is unknown, send bloods for paracetamol levels, autoantibody screen and hepatitis viral screen (Hep A, B, C, EBV, CMV, HSV). Consider sending blood for copper and caeruloplasmin levels. Do a pregnancy test in women of childbearing age.
- Insert a urinary catheter and send urine for microscopy and culture.
- Get a chest X-ray.
- If ascites is present, perform a diagnostic ascitic tap and send for urgent cell count and microscopy. If the neutrophil count is > 250 per mm^3, treat for spontaneous bacterial peritonitis (check local protocols but treat with broad spectrum antibiotics e.g. ceftriaxone 2 g IV od).
- Order an urgent ultrasound scan of the liver (looking for size, biliary tree obstruction and venous outflow obstruction).

General management

- Start a dextrose infusion; if BM < 4, give 50 mL 50% dextrose and then a 10% dextrose infusion; otherwise give 5% dextrose. Add potassium and magnesium if needed to correct electrolytes.
- Start lactulose 30 mL three times per day. Reduce the dose once diarrhoea starts.
- Give intravenous B-complex vitamins (Pabrinex), plus thiamine and folic acid. Give 10 mg of vitamin K intravenously.

- If paracetamol overdose is the likely cause, give intravenous *N*-acetylcysteine, even if > 24 h since the overdose.
- Avoid sedative drugs and medications with hepatic metabolism (see the BNF for details).
- Nurse in a high-dependency area, with hourly pulse, BP, urine output and neurological observations.

Hypoglycaemia Give 10% dextrose infusion. Give a bolus of 50 mL of 50% dextrose if BM < 4.

Hypotension Insert a central line (get help with this) because the INR is likely to be elevated. Give albumin or colloid; avoid giving saline. Give blood for GI bleeding or if anaemic. If still hypotensive despite an adequate CVP, inotropic support is needed; discuss with your senior.

Poor urine output/renal failure This could be due to sepsis, dehydration, GI bleeding or hepatorenal failure. Exclude the first three (insert a central line and rehydrate) and enlist expert help; a combination of terlipressin and albumin might improve hepatorenal failure.

Coma A reduced GCS suggests high-grade hepatic encephalopathy. Intubation and ventilation on ITU are probably needed. Talk to your seniors immediately. A sudden deterioration might be due to intracranial bleeding or fits.

Fitting Treat along standard lines (see 'Fits' and 'Status epilepticus', pp. 176, 108).

Bacterial peritonitis Treat with intravenous antibiotics, e.g. ciprofloxacin/ceftriaxone. If fever is present without an obvious focus, treat with broad-spectrum antibiotics.

Ascites Treat with spironolactone or, if massive, by paracentesis. Discuss with your senior; treatment of ascites can be difficult in the presence of low sodium or haemodynamic instability. Drain fluid should be replaced with albumin at a rate of 1 unit for every 2 L ascitic fluid drained. The drain should be removed at 6 h to reduce the risk of infection.

Low sodium If the patient is fluid overloaded, fluid restrict to 1 L/day. Stop diuretics if sodium is < 125 mmol/L. If the patient is not fluid overloaded, discuss with a hepatologist.

Points to watch

- Discuss all patients with decompensated liver disease with a hepatologist. The earlier such patients are seen, the earlier they can be transferred to ITU and/or a transplant unit if necessary.
- Signs that all is not well are:
  - persistent hypotension
  - persistent metabolic acidosis
  - worsening renal failure
  - declining GCS.
- Do not correct clotting abnormalities with FFP unless: (i) the patient is bleeding; or (ii) you need to carry out an invasive procedure. The INR is one of the best markers of hepatic synthetic function, and correction with FFP negates its usefulness.

Upper GI bleed

Diagnosis

By the presence of red vomitus (haematemesis) or melaena. Coffee ground vomit is not always due to GI bleeding; consider normal foodstuffs and obstruction as well. GI bleeds should be managed on a GI bleed unit or high-dependency unit.

What to do

- Put in two large-bore cannulae (16G or above). Take blood for FBC, group and save, U+Es, LFTs and clotting.
- Take a quick history, looking especially for a history of alcohol abuse, liver disease, NSAID use.
- Examine the patient, looking especially for the pulse, BP both lying and sitting or standing, signs of liver disease including asterixis and confusion. A PR exam is mandatory.
- Start an IV infusion. If the patient has no history of liver disease, this should be saline. In patients with a history of liver disease, use 5% dextrose.
- If the patient has a systolic BP < 100, give 500 mL of colloid as quickly as possible and ask the lab for an urgent cross-match for 4 units. Do not wait for the FBC result. Repeat the colloid infusion if BP still < 100.
- If the systolic BP is > 100 but the pulse is > 100 per min, or there is a postural BP drop of > 20 mmHg, run in fluids at 1 L/h until the tachycardia or postural drop resolves.
- Features of a significant bleed include: Age > 60, systolic BP < 100 mmHg, heart rate > 100 bpm, chronic liver disease, significant comorbidity (lung, heart, renal disease), Hb < 10 g/l
- If there are features of a significant bleed (e.g. by Blatchford or Rockall's score), call your senior and consider the use of IV proton pump inhibitor (PPI) depending on your local guidelines.
- If a variceal bleed is suspected, consider the use of IV PPI and IV terlipressin (2 mg IV bolus followed by 2 mg IV 6 hourly).
- Monitor pulse, BP and urine output every hour, more frequently if BP is low. If the urine output is poor, or BP is still low after 1 L of colloid, insert a CVP line. Also consider inserting a CVP line if you suspect a variceal bleed.
- If urine is not passed within 3–4 h, or if BP is low, insert a urinary catheter.

GIVING BLOOD

- If a patient is exsanguinating in front of you, call you senior and get someone to fetch O negative blood from the blood fridge. Give this as fast as possible. If the patient is shocked, give blood without waiting for the FBC.
- If the patient is not shocked, transfuse over a period of several hours, aiming for an Hb of 10 g/dL (1 unit roughly equals 1 g/dL).
- If clotting is deranged, administer IV vitamin K, together with either FFP or clotting factor concentrate (D-fix).

Endoscopy Consult your local protocol. If stable and non-variceal, endoscopy can usually be performed in the morning, once transfused. If shocked or rebleeding, try and resuscitate first. If bleeding is torrential, emergency endoscopy (sometimes even at the bedside) might be required. Suspected variceal bleeds should be endoscoped urgently (ideally within 4 h). Resuscitate the patient before endoscopy if at all possible.

Surgery Inform the on-call surgical team of any significant bleed. Tell them again if a patient rebleeds after having been stable.

Points to watch

- Patients with an acute GI bleed do not drop their haemoglobin levels immediately; it takes several hours for haemodilution to occur. A normal haemoglobin does not exclude a GI bleed.
- Older patients, or those on rate-limiting agents (e.g. beta-blockers), cannot produce a tachycardic response to hypovolaemia. They thus tend to suffer hypotension after relatively small losses.
- Conversely, young patients can suffer a large blood loss before decompensating and dropping their blood pressure; hence a normal blood pressure does not exclude a significant bleed.

Points to note with variceal bleeds

- Suspect in anyone with signs of chronic liver disease
- Insert a central line; aggressive fluid and blood replacement is needed, but overfilling increases portal pressure and might precipitate a rebleed
- GI bleeds can precipitate hepatic encephalopathy
- Correct clotting abnormalities vigorously with FFP and vitamin K
- Commence IV PPI and IV Terlipressin
- Inform the endoscopist as soon as possible – do not wait until the morning. Variceal bleeds require urgent endoscopy

---

Rockall's score

Variable	score			
	0	1	2	3
Age (years)	<60	60–79	≥80	
Shock	Pulse <100 Systolic bp > 100 mmHg	Pulse ≥ 100 bpm Systolic Bp ≥ 100 mmHg	Bp ≤ 100 mmHg	
Comorbidity	No major comorbidity		Cardiac disease, ischaemic heart disease, any major co-morbidity	Renal failure, liver failure, disseminated malignancy
Diagnosis	Mallory Weiss tear, no lesion identified and SRH/blood	All other diagnoses	Malignancy of upper GI tract	
Major stigmata of major GI haemorrhage	None or dark spot only		Blood in upper GI tract, adherent clot visible or spurting vessel	
Examples of comorbidity	No or mild co-existing illness (e.g. ECG abnormalities without symptoms)	Moderate co-existing illnessess (e.g. hypertension stable with medication)	Severe coexisting illnesses (diseases requiring immediate treatment e.g. cardiac failure)	Life-threatening diseases (e.g. end-stage malignancy, renal failure)

(Modified from Vreeburg et al. *Gut* 1999; 44:331–335)

Predicted probabilities		
Risk score	Rebleeding (%)	Mortality (%)
0	4.9	0
1	3.4	0
2	5.3	0.2
3	11.2	2.9
4	14.1	5.3
5	24.1	10.8
6	32.9	17.3
7	43.8	27.0
8+	41.8	31.1
Total	18.9	10.0

Acute renal failure

Diagnosis

A rapidly rising creatinine and urea. Acute renal failure is accompanied by oliguria (< 400 mL/24 h) in 80% of cases.

What to do

- Take a history and examine the patient. The history is the key to eliciting the cause of the renal failure; the examination will give clues as to the hydration state of the patient. The drug history in particular is often of paramount importance.

- Take blood for U+Es, FBC, calcium, phosphate, CK, glucose, CRP, ESR and autoimmune screen (ANA, RF, complement, ANCA, anti-GBM), along with hepatitis serology. Take urgent arterial blood gases and establish IV access.

MANAGING HYPERKALAEMIA

- If the potassium is > 7, emergency measures are required to bring it down:
  - give 10 mL of 10% calcium gluconate. This does not reduce the potassium level; it merely stabilizes the electrical state of the cardiac myocytes
  - attach an ECG monitor
  - give Insulin/Dextrose (10 units Actrapid/Velosulin in 50 mL 50% Dextrose over 20 min)
- Perform an ECG. If tenting of the T waves is present, follow the above protocol.
- If the potassium is 6.0–6.9 without ECG changes, attach an ECG monitor and give insulin and dextrose as above.
- If the potassium is 5.0–5.9, stop drugs that cause hyperkalaemia (e.g. ACE inhibitors, spironolactone) and ensure a low-potassium diet.

Managing fluid balance Insert a urinary catheter and attach to a urometer to closely monitor output. A CVP line may be helpful to assess the patients hydration status.

If the CVP is low, give a bolus of 250–500 mL fluid over 15 min. If the CVP fails to rise, or rises only transiently, repeat until CVP rises. If the CVP is high, do not administer any fluids. If the CVP is intermediate, give a 250-mL bolus of fluid as above.

Treating acidosis Consult a renal physician urgently if there is profound acidosis; dialysis is often a better method of dealing with this problem than the administration of bicarbonate.

TREATING THE UNDERLYING CAUSE

- Obtain an urgent ultrasound of the kidneys, especially if the patient is anuric and if serum creatinine > 400 mmol/L. Obstruction of only one kidney can cause acute renal failure if the other kidney functions poorly.

- Treat sepsis; look for a source. If blood pressure remains low despite a high CVP, commence inotropic support such as dobutamine and will need to be on a high dependency unit.

OTHER SUPPORTIVE TREATMENT

- Stop all nephrotoxic drugs, e.g. furosemide (frusemide), aminoglycosides, ACE inhibitors, NSAIDs. Stop any drugs that could accumulate and cause further problems, e.g. metformin, digoxin.
- There is no evidence to support using renal-dose dopamine, especially in established acute renal failure.

Points to watch

- Is it acute or chronic renal failure? Try and find some old notes or blood results. The presence of hyperkalaemia or acidosis suggests acute renal failure. The presence of normocytic anaemia suggests chronic renal failure, but acute renal failure might supervene.
- Urine output versus renal failure: 20% of patients with acute renal failure have non-oliguric renal failure. Look at the bloods, not just the urine output.
- Not everyone with oliguria has renal failure. Most patients excrete less urine overnight and older people, especially women of small stature, have relatively low urine outputs; 750–1000 mL in 24 h is not uncommon. Such individuals might have a urine output of < 30 mL/h for several hours overnight.

When to dialyse

In general, involve the renal physicians early – especially if you do not have dialysis on site. Absolute indications for dialysis include: • refractory fluid overload • profound acidosis • refractory hyperkalaemia • severe uraemia (e.g. causing fits, pericarditis or reduced conscious level) • ARF unresponsive to conservative therapy

In general, there is a move towards dialysing earlier rather than later in the course of acute renal failure, so as to avoid the complications of acidosis, high potassium and uraemia

Acute asthma

Diagnosis

Patients with asthma are usually young and present with breathlessness and wheeze. If you suspect asthma, stop and think 'Is this COPD?'. Asthmatics are usually young, have had asthma since childhood and have little or no smoking history. Late-onset asthma is less common. Patients with COPD are older, have late-onset symptoms and almost always have a significant smoking history.

Differential diagnosis of the breathless patient

- Exacerbation of COPD • Pneumonia • Left ventricular failure • Pnuemothorax
- Pulmonary embolism

What to do

- Assess the patient quickly – check ABC. Make sure the airway is patent, check that the vital signs are stable and examine the patient's chest.
- Assess for the following features in particular:
  - severe asthma: cannot complete sentences in one breath; respiratory rate > 25 breaths/min; pulse > 110 bpm; PEFR 33–50% best/predicted
  - life-threatening signs: silent chest/feeble respiratory effort; bradycardia/ hypotension; exhaustion; confusion/coma; PEFR < 33% predicted.
- If any of the latter features appear, call for senior help urgently; the patient is minutes away from a cardiorespiratory arrest.
- Give high flow O_2 using a non-rebreath bag.
- Give 5 mg nebulized salbutamol and 500 µg nebulized Ipratropium with O_2 as the driving gas.
- If patient is able to swallow, give 30–40 mg prednisolone PO. If not, give 100–200 mg hydrocortisone IV.
- Perform an arterial blood gas. Patients with a low pO_2 (< 8 kPa) or a normal or high pCO_2 (4–6 kPa) are at high risk.

If patient displays severe or life-threatening features with no improvement with initial therapy, give IV magnesium (1.2–2 g over 20 min)

- Get a chest X-ray to exclude pneumothorax or pneumonia. Routine antibiotic use is not indicated.
- Do routine bloods, including aminophylline levels and blood cultures if appropriate.
- If there is no improvement, get help. Consider using aminophylline by giving 250 mg (5 mg/kg) over 15–20 min followed by an infusion of 0.5 mg/kg/h. ECG monitoring is required. Caution is needed if the patient is already on theophyllines – omit the bolus dose.

Points to watch

ABGs and O_2 therapy in asthma Patients with asthma do not retain CO_2 routinely. If they do, they are very unwell and the CO_2 retention is a result of hypoventilation (due to exhaustion) and hence poor gas exchange. Asthmatics do not depend on hypoxia for their ventilatory drive. These patients need mechanical ventilation.

Some patients with COPD retain CO_2 chronically and the mechanism is different – they come to depend on hypoxia for their ventilatory drive, hence high-dose O_2 is potentially dangerous. Examples of ABGs seen in asthma are given in Fig. 32.

MILD–MODERATE ASTHMA

- Most attacks of asthma that are seen will be mild to moderate in severity; mild = PEFR >75% predicted; moderate = PEFR 50–75% predicted.
- Give normal inhalers if mild asthma. Observe for 1 h.
- Repeat PEFR. If:
  - >75% predicted PEFR, then discharge home
  - 50–75% then give nebulizers (salbutamol and ipratropium), 30–40 mg prednisolone orally.
- Repeat PEFR 30 min later. If:
  - >75%, discharge with inhaled steroids
  - 50–75%, observe for further 1 h and if not improved, admit
  - <50% predicted, admit for observation, nebulizers, steroids, ABGs, chest X-ray and O_2.

MODERATE ASTHMA

Treat initially with nebulizers and steroids and recheck peak flow at 1 h. If < 75%, admit for observation, nebulizers, steroids, blood gases and chest X-ray (British Thoracic Society and Scottish Intercollegiate Guidelines Network. Guidelines for the Management of Asthma. April 2004).

> ### Hints
> If the patient is unwell and not improving, it is better to treat aggressively and quickly. Call for senior help if you are at all worried – asthmatics can deteriorate rapidly.

Typical ABGs in asthma		
pH 7.45	pH 7.1	pH 7.35
pO_2 27.6	pO_2 11.1	pO_2 12.2
pCO_2 2.9	pCO_2 7.1	pCO_2 5.0
Typical acute asthma	Life-threatening asthma	Severe asthma (beginning to tire)
On O_2 hence high pO_2	CO_2 retention and acidosis	Normal CO_2 and O_2
Hyperventilating and blowing off CO_2	This is peri-arrest	Look at the patient!

Fig. 32 Examples of typical arterial blood gases (ABGs) in asthma.

Acute exacerbation of COPD

Diagnosis

Patients with COPD present more commonly to hospital than asthmatics. They are older and usually have a strong smoking history (usually 10–20 cigarettes a day for >20 years). Diagnosis is on the basis of increased wheeze and shortness of breath, accompanied by increased volume and/or increased purulence of sputum.

What to do

- Assess the patient, especially the vital signs, including GCS, respiratory rate and O_2 saturations. Exclude upper airway obstruction. Confusion, exhaustion, reduced level of consciousness or low blood pressure are all signs of a life-threatening attack. If any of these features are present, call for senior help.

- Examine the patient quickly looking for signs of poor inspiratory effort, wheeze, consolidation or pulmonary oedema.

- Treat with 24–28% O_2 and do baseline ABGs after 30 min of treatment.

- Give 5 mg salbutamol and 500 µg ipratropium bromide through an air-driven nebulizer. Give 2 L O_2 via nasal prongs if necessary.

- Give 30–40 mg prednisolone PO (or 100–200 mg IV hydrocortisone if unable to swallow).

- Repeat nebulizers. If no improvement, the patient may need non-invasive ventilation. Contact your senior. Consider aminophylline treatment if not improving (250–500 mg over 15–20 min if not on oral therapy, followed by an infusion of 0.5 mg/kg/min).

- Monitor ABGs regularly, especially when titrating O_2 therapy. Usually this should by done hourly but it might have to be done more frequently if the patient's conscious level or O_2 saturations fall (see below).

- Get a chest X-ray to look for infection, pulmonary oedema and pneumothorax.

- Perform a 12-lead ECG because patients can be in uncontrolled atrial fibrillation/flutter, which should be treated with digoxin. Salbutamol can also lower K^+ and can trigger arrhythmias, as can aminophylline infusions, which should therefore be subject to cardiac monitoring.

- Try to get a history from the patient or relatives. Look for features suggesting an acute exacerbation. These include worsening of a previously stable condition, e.g. reduced exercise tolerance, increased wheeze, breathlessness, sputum production and sputum purulence. Also ask about chest tightness and ankle swelling.

- Other important features in the history include the normal condition including exercise tolerance, presence of home nebulizers or O_2, the number of previous hospital admissions for exacerbations including number of admissions requiring ventilation, and the smoking history. Seriously question the diagnosis if there is no history of smoking.

Points to watch

COPD, CO_2, and O_2 therapy Many patients with COPD have chronically high CO_2 levels and chronically low O_2 levels. In acute exacerbations, however, the pH will indicate whether this rise in CO_2 is chronic or acute. If it is normal, the chronic hypercapnia will have been compensated for; a low pH suggests an acute rise in CO_2 because there is little time for compensation.

During acute exacerbations, aim for a pO_2 of ≥ 8 kPa. Titrate the O_2 up from 24% to 28% in steps (35%, 40%, 50%, 60–80%), until this level is reached without an increase in CO_2. If the CO_2 does begin to rise, with inadequate oxygenation, the patient should be considered for ventilation. Equally, if the patient is acidotic (pH < 7.3), then the patient should be considered for ventilation. The usual method for ventilation nowadays is non-invasive ventilation (NIV) given via a tight-fitting facemask, rather than via an endotracheal tube; this can be quickly started in high-dependency areas outside of the ITU. Some examples of ABGs seen in COPD are given in Fig. 33.

Antibiotics in COPD

Think of infection if: • there is a history of worsening sputum production/purulence • there is a history of bronchiectasis • there is chest pain • temperature > 38°C

If you are suspicious of an infection, commence oral antibiotics (amoxicillin 500 mg three times per day or erythromycin 500 mg four times per day if penicillin allergic). If life-threatening features appear, give IV antibiotics, e.g. cefuroxime 750 mg three times per day. Check your local guidelines for your hospital policy. (British Thoracic Society guidelines. *Thorax* 1997; 52 suppl 5:S1–S32.)

Guide to non-invasive ventilation

Patients should be considered for NIV with acute acidotic exacerbations (pH < 7.35 and $pCO_2 > 6.0$ kPa).
Use a full fitting face mask.
Start NIV at EPAP + 4 cm and IPAP +10 cm Increase IPAP by 2 over the next 1 hour to maximum of +20 cm or whatever is best tolerated.
Set ventilator to timed.
Aim for 1–2 L O_2 with sats 85–90%.
Repeat ABGs after 1 hour
If ABGs worsen, consider for ITU and invasive ventilation.

Typical ABGs in COPD	
pH 7.4	pH 7.1
pCO_2 7.0	pCO_2 7.9
pO_2 9.1	pO_2 7.5
Probably normal for this patient	Type II respiratory failure
Chronic compensated ↑CO_2	↓pH with acute CO_2 retention and hypoxia
Mild hypoxia and normal pH	Call for help

Fig. 33 Examples of typical arterial blood gases (ABGs) in chronic obstructive pulmonary disease COPD.

Pulmonary embolism

Diagnosis

Think of pulmonary embolism (PE) in any patient who presents with breathlessness or pleuritic chest pain. It can be missed in the elderly, patients with known cardio-respiratory disease (e.g. COPD) and in patients who present only with breathless-ness. Major risks for PE include:

- Patients having undergone recent surgery (major abdominal/pelvic surgery, hip/ knee replacement).
- Prolonged immobility (e.g. institutional care, prolonged hospitalization).
- Patients with a major medical illness, e.g. abdominal/pelvic/disseminated malignancy.
- Pregnancy or postpartum.
- Lower limb problems (fractures/varicose veins).
- Patients with previously proven DVT/PE.

Minor risks include:

- Patients with a history of long-distance travel.
- Previous history of thrombophilia or strong family history of thromboembolic disease.
- Patients on the oral contraceptive pill or HRT are often referred but this is considered a minor risk factor.

> ### Differential diagnosis for patients presenting with pleuritic chest pain:
> • Pneumonia • Pulmonary embolism • Pneumothorax • Musculoskeletal pain (e.g. muscle tear, costochondritis) • Pericarditis

What to do

- Look for life-threatening features: uncontrolled tachycardia (HR > 120 bpm), collapse/hypotension (BP < 90 mmHg systolic), respiratory rate > 30 per min, hypoxia (pO_2 < 8 kPa). If any of these features occur, call your senior; the patient might need thrombolysis.
- Assess the patient rapidly, looking for features of alternative diagnosis, e.g. tension pneumothorax, upper airways obstruction.
- Give O_2 at 60–80% via a non-rebreathing (reservoir) bag.
- Insert a large cannula into a peripheral vein and send off bloods for FBC, U+Es, CRP, glucose, CK and clotting. Give 250 mL IV colloid if the patient is hypotensive.
- Attach the patient to a cardiac monitor.
- Get an urgent chest X-ray and 12-lead ECG. Do an arterial blood gas.
- If the patient has life-threatening features, try and confirm the diagnosis via either:

- a CT Pulmonary Angiogram (CTPA) – probably the most readily available in emergencies or
- an echocardiogram – useful to look for right heart strain but also to exclude aortic dissection, pericardial tamponade and myocardial infarction.

- Some kind of investigation should be performed to confirm the diagnosis of PE and appropriate treatment given – the exception is obviously when the patient is periarrest where clinical judgement is crucial. If the above investigations suggest pulmonary embolism, consider thrombolytic therapy – discuss with your senior.

If no features of haemodynamic compromise are present:

- Take a history, looking particularly for major risk factors. Patients can present with a wide spectrum of symptoms ranging from sudden collapse with chest pain, to haemoptysis, pleuritic chest pain or isolated breathlessness. It is unusual for patients to present with a PE without breathlessness. It is also unusual to be the correct diagnosis in the absence of breathlessness or tachypnoea (RR > 20/min).

- Examine the patient looking for other reasons for their symptoms, e.g. consolidation, or confirmatory signs, e.g. a raised JVP.

- Take bloods if not already done, and perform blood gases on air. If clinical suspicion of PE is high (i.e. in the presence of significant risk-factors for PE), then D-dimer testing should NOT be performed. If, however, there is a low or intermediate clinical risk of PE, then a negative D-dimer may be helpful in excluding a PE without imaging.

- Perform a chest X-ray to exclude other pathology, e.g. pneumothorax, pneumonia.

- CTPA has now superseded V/Q scanning as the most common investigation for non-life-threatening PE, but some centres may still use perfusion scans in patients with normal chest X-rays.

- Pulmonary angiography – the gold-standard test for a PE but is very rarely performed.

- Give 40–60% O_2.

- Start anticoagulation with heparin:
    - low-molecular-weight heparin (as per local guidelines)
    - unfractionated heparin in patients in whom there may be a risk of bleeding (e.g. post-operatively): 5000 U bolus followed by 24 000 U over 24 h. Ensure APTTr is measured at 4–6 h and is maintained at 1.5–2.5

- After confirmation of the diagnosis, patients should be anticoagulated with warfarin for at least 6 months with a target INR of 2–3 (3–4 if recurrent PEs). If a PE is confirmed with no obvious risk factors, look for an underlying cause, e.g. occult malignancy, thrombophilia (see 'The swollen leg' p. 180, for more details).

Points to watch

- Typical ABGs with a pulmonary embolism are shown in Fig. 34. The most common picture is of hypoxia with mild respiratory alkalosis due to appropriate hyperventilation. Remember that blood gases might be normal following a small peripheral embolism.

Typical ABGs in PE	
pH	7.5
pO_2	8.0
pCO_2	3.1

Fig. 34 Typical arterial blood gases (ABGs) in pulmonary embolism (PE).

- 12-lead ECG: usually shows sinus tachycardia but look for right axis deviation, right bundle branch block or signs of right heart strain. $S_IQ_{III}T_{III}$ (deep S wave in lead I, Q wave and inverted T wave in lead III) occurs in people without PE and is of little diagnostic value.

- D-dimers: negative D-dimers make the diagnosis of PE very unlikely in patients with a low or intermediate clinical risk of PE. Positive D-dimers could be due to PE but also to DVT, MI, sepsis, trauma or other acute inflammatory conditions. Patients with a high clinical risk of PE (i.e. in the presence of major risk factors for PE) should procede directly to imaging without D-dimer measurement. (British Thoracic Society guidelines. *Thorax* 2003; 58:470–484.)

Pneumonia

Diagnosis

Commonly presents with pleuritic chest pain, fever and cough. However, elderly patients can present with less specific symptoms, such as collapse, confusion or 'off-legs'. The most common organism is still *Streptococcus pneumoniae*, which is usually sensitive to penicillin.

What to do

- ABC – ensure the patient's airway is patent and check all vital signs: pulse, blood pressure, respiratory rate and O_2 saturations. Assess the pneumonia severity (CURB-65 score) and document this in the notes.

- If the patient is hypotensive (< 90 mmHg systolic or < 60 mmHg diastolic) call for senior help – your patient might be in septic shock. Obtain IV access via a large peripheral vein with a wide-bore cannula and give 500 mL of IV colloid over 10–20 min. If the patient is elderly or has a history of heart failure, reduce the rate and the amount infused.

- If O_2 saturations are < 95%, perform arterial blood gases and give appropriate O_2 therapy (40–60%) to maintain saturations above 92%. Be careful with O_2 therapy in patients with known COPD.

- Take a history, looking for features of previous lung disease, smoking history and any other significant comorbidity. Examine the patient for signs of consolidation and any other cause for breathlessness, e.g. pneumothorax, pulmonary oedema.

- Obtain a chest X-ray to confirm consolidation and to assess severity, e.g. bilateral and multilobar pneumonia.

- Perform an ECG – pneumonia can cause AF or atrial flutter, especially in elderly patients. This often resolves with treatment of the underlying infection. Look for evidence of ischaemia.

- Send routine bloods: FBC, U+Es, LFTs, CRP and blood cultures. Send a 10 mL clotted sample for atypical serology. If *Legionella* infection is suspected, send off a urine specimen for antigen testing as well as urine for pneumococcal antigen testing in severe pneumonia.

- Give IV fluids to maintain hydration and treat sepsis – patients with fever have higher than normal insensible losses and may not drink enough to cover them and in younger patients aggressive fluid management in the presence of sepsis improves outcome.

- If no features of severe pneumonia exist, give oral antibiotics. Ensure blood cultures have been sent. Check with your local antibiotic policy; amoxicillin 500 mg tds plus a macrolide (use erythromycin 500 mg four times per day) is a good starting point.

- If any features of severity are present (eg CURB-65 score of 2 or more), call your senior. Give intravenous antibiotics (e.g. IV co-amoxiclav 1.2 g or cefuroxime 750 mg 8-hourly; check your local prescribing policy) and treatment with a macrolide (erythromycin or clarithromycin IV).

- Check the ECG. If the patient is in AF or atrial flutter, load with digoxin for rate control (see 'Arrhythmias', p. 103). The AF often resolves with treatment of the underlying infection.

If pleurisy is present, give analgesis (eg NSAIDs).

Assessment of community-acquired pneumonia (CURB-65 score)

Confusion/reduced level of consciousness
  serum Urea > 7 mmol/L
Respiratory rate > 30/min
  systolic BP < 90 mmHg $\pm$ diastolic BP < 60 mmHg
  age $\geq$ 65 years old
CURB-65 Score 0 or 1 – low risk of death; could be managed at home
CURB-65 Score 2 – should be treated in hospital and considered for HDU
CURB-65 Score > 3 more – higher risk of death. Should be managed as severe pneumonia on HDU/ITU

Additional clinical adverse prognostic features:
- hypoxaemia: pO_2 < 8 kPa
- bilateral or multilobar changes on chest X-ray

Points to watch

Monitor the clinical state, temperature, WCC and CRP. If these do not settle consider the following:

- Wrong antibiotics: most pneumococci are sensitive to penicillin, but confirm the organism and sensitivities with your microbiology lab. TB is becoming more common and must be considered, especially in patients from the Indian subcontinent. Consider also infections related to HIV/AIDS and other immunocompromised conditions, e.g. *Staphylococcus* and *Cryptococcus* infection.

- Empyema: any patient developing a pleural effusion related to the infection must have an urgent diagnostic pleural tap performed and pH checked. If pus is found or if the fluid pH is < 7.2, senior and specialist help should be sought because the patient has an empyema or complicated parapneumonic effusion and this must be drained. A fluid pH of > 7.2 (a simple parapneumonic effusion) needs close monitoring.

- Wrong diagnosis: consider pulmonary infarction and pulmonary oedema. Bronchial carcinoma might also be present and can coexist with the pneumonia preventing resolution. Bronchoscopy may be required.

Hospital-acquired pneumonia

Organisms causing pneumonia in hospital can be different from the ones in the community. Local guidelines should be checked but there tend to be more penicillin-resistant strains in hospital so other treatments should be considered, e.g. co-amoxiclav 625 mg three times a day.

Aspiration pneumonia

Aspiration pneumonia occurs in patients with swallowing difficulties and a history of unconsciousness or vomiting. Include anaerobic cover, e.g. cefuroxime plus metronidazole, or co-amoxiclav.

(British Thoracic Society guidelines – 2004 Update. www.brit-thoracic.org/guidelines).

Pneumothorax

Diagnosis

Spontaneous pneumothorax occurs classically in young, tall, thin men, although it also occurs in patients with pre-existing lung disease, e.g. asthma, COPD. Procedure-related pnuemothoraces occur not uncommonly after subclavian line insertion, pleural biopsy and permanent pacemaker insertion.

Think of this diagnosis in young, previously healthy patients presenting with sudden onset pleuritic chest pain and breathlessness.

What to do

- If the patient presents with a pneumothorax and BP < 90 mmHg, suspect a tension pneumothorax. A patient who is haemodynamically compromised is about to arrest:
  - insert a large cannula into the second intercostal space in the midclavicular line on the side of reduced breath sounds. If there is a tension pneumothorax, the air will rush out and blood pressure will improve. Insert a chest drain immediately.

- If the patient is haemodynamically stable, give O_2 to maintain O_2 saturation > 95% (be cautious in patients with COPD).

- Take a history, including details of previous pnuemothoraces and their side, pre-existing lung disease, smoking history and previous lung surgery.

- Perform a chest X-ray to confirm the diagnosis. If the X-ray looks normal, check the apices and right heart border and obtain inspiratory films.

- In patients with no history of lung disease, needle-aspirate the affected lung and try to remove as much air as possible. Repeat the chest X-ray to assess progress. If the lung has reinflated fully, repeat the chest X-ray at 7 days to confirm reinflation. Ask the patient to avoid air travel and to return if there is any deterioration of symptoms. If the lung has partially reinflated, consider reaspiration and maintain on O_2. If the lung has not reinflated, insert a chest drain.

- In patients with existing lung disease, small apical pneumothoraces can be managed conservatively and with O_2. However, if there is a moderate or large pneumothorax, a chest drain should be inserted to prevent respiratory compromise.

- See 'Chest drain insertion' and 'Chest drain removal' (p. 78) for details of how to manage a chest drain.

Surgical emergencies

The acute abdomen

The vast majority of surgical emergencies involve the assessment of patients with an acute abdomen. The diagnosis is made on history, examination and key investigations.

What to do

- Check ABC.
- Look for signs of haemodynamic compromise: BP < 90 mmHg systolic, pulse > 110/min, drowsiness, sweating, pallor, capillary refill > 2 s, poor urine output.
- If any of these features appear, the patient might be in shock and you should call for senior help.
- Resuscitate the patient:
  - give O_2 via non-rebreathe mask
  - get IV access – try for two large-bore cannulae, one in each antecubital fossa
  - take blood for FBC, U+Es, cross-match 4 units of blood
  - take blood cultures and arterial blood gases.
- Examine the patient, looking for signs of infection or blood loss.
- If the patient is haemodynamically stable, you have more time for a formal assessment.
- Give analgesia. Patients are quite often in pain when they present to hospital. The key to making the diagnosis is the ability to assess the patient accurately. This cannot be done if the patient is in pain. For severe pain, give 5–10 mg morphine IV plus 50 mg cyclizine IV. For suspected renal colic give 100 mg diclofenac rectally.

HISTORY
Take a full history of the pain once the patient is comfortable.

- Pain described as gripping in nature, periodic and occurring in 'waves' is colic and means a hollow viscus may be obstructed.
- Pain that is better localized and is made worse by coughing or moving ('the journey into hospital was awful, I felt every bump in the road') suggests peritonitis.

EXAMINATION
Check vital signs including temperature. The abdomen is divided into sections, each of which corresponds to different organs (see 'Abdominal examination', p. 232). Ask the patient to lie completely flat and point with one finger to the area of maximum pain. Examine the patient's abdomen beginning away from the most painful area. Tenderness to percussion equals peritonism. Always check for bowel sounds and do not forget to do a rectal examination.

Dipstick urine for blood and protein. Perform a pregnancy test on all premenopausal women.

INVESTIGATIONS
- All patients should have a cannula inserted. Take blood samples for FBC, U+Es, LFTs, amylase, CRP and group and save in all patients.
- Check INR if you suspect liver disease or sepsis.

- X-rays should be performed for a reason – a young person with suspected appendicitis needs no X-rays. An abdominal X-ray is needed in patients with suspected obstruction to look for dilation, in renal colic (KUB/CTKUB dependent on departmental policy), pancreatitis and in patients in whom the diagnosis is still unknown. A chest X-ray is needed for diagnositic reasons (has the patient perforated a viscus) or anaesthetic reasons (known respiratory comorbidity and needs an operation). Someone walking around the surgical admission ward without signs of peritonitis does not need a chest X-ray.
- Take blood cultures if the patient has a fever > 38°C.
- Any patient who is suspected of serious bleeding, e.g. ruptured ectopic pregnancy, ruptured AAA, should have 8 units of blood cross-matched. If you suspect a patient will require a laparotomy, electronic cross match should suffice. Check your local protocol however; these amounts are a guide only.

OTHER POINTS

Nil by mouth All patients with a surgical abdomen or who might need theatre should be kept nil by mouth; 6 h nil by mouth are needed to safely empty the gut for general anaesthesia. Normal oral medication should still be taken with a sip of water

Fluids
- Patients who present with a surgical abdomen are almost always dehydrated and should be prescribed IV fluids. Most patients under the age of 70 should be given 1 L IV normal saline over 4 h followed by litre bags over 6 and 8 h. If the patient is unwell, 1 L of fluid should be given stat, with further fluid given over 1, 2, 4 and 6 h.
- Be cautious in patients with known heart failure and in the elderly, but ensure that fluid replacement is adequate; renal failure is harder to treat than fluid overload.
- Most surgical patients are intravascularly dry and leaking plasma: give normal saline alone initially and add potassium only after the results are known.
- Patients with diabetes should be put on an IV sliding scale of insulin with hourly BMs and a combination of normal saline and 5% dextrose depending on their blood sugars (use dextrose if BM < 10).

Drug chart Patients should have all of their normal medication prescribed. Diabetics on sliding scales should have their normal insulin and oral hypoglycaemics omitted; any patient who is hypotensive should obviously have their antihypertensive medication stopped. Medications can be given with a sip of water even if nil by mouth.

Prescribe adequate analgesia with appropriate antiemetics, e.g. diamorphine 5–10 mg IV and cyclizine 50 mg IV/PO/IM.

DVT prophylaxis

All patients should have TED stockings and most will need prophylactic heparin (omit in anyone presenting with bleeding). However, this should not be given to someone who is about to go to theatre and will need an epidural catheter as this cannot be inserted if heparin has been given recently.

Acute appendicitis

A very common cause for a surgical admission. Appendicitis can kill – treat it with respect.

Diagnosis

Right iliac fossa pain, worsening with time, should be assumed to be possible appendicitis, especially if it is accompanied by guarding and rebound tenderness, raised WCC or fever.

What to do

- Take a history. The usual history is of 1–2 days of central vague abdominal pain localizing to the right iliac fossa. Pain is usually constant with associated nausea and vomiting. Appendicitis can present atypically, e.g. right hypochondrium in pregnancy, diarrhoea in retrocaecal appendix. In women, take a gynaecological history – previous history, surgery, LMP, irregular bleeding/discharge. It is uncommon to feel hungry with appendicitis.
- Examine the patient. Patients usually have mild fever (around 37.5°C) although they can be afebrile. There is usually right iliac fossa tenderness with guarding and rebound. Rectal examination is usually tender, particularly on the right side. Patients who can walk around do not usually have florid appendicitis. Look at the chest, ears, nose and throat for alternative diagnoses.
- Investigations: WCC might be elevated slightly, although it can also be normal. Check urine dipstick for blood/protein. A pregnancy test in all premenopausal women is mandatory.
- There is no point in performing X-rays on a patient with appendicitis unless you suspect another cause for the pain, e.g. obstruction.
- Blood cultures if fever > 37.5°C is present.
- Management: keep patient NBM and give IV fluids. Give adequate analgesia and antiemetics and get your seniors to review for surgery.

Differential diagnosis

- Mesenteric adenitis – particularly in children with recent illness.
- Gynaecological causes: infection, ruptured ectopic pregnancy, ruptured ovarian cyst.
- Urinary tract infection.
- Ruptured ulcer or caecum (e.g. caecal carcinoma).
- Inflammatory bowel disease.
- Diverticulitis.
- Infective enterocolitis.

Ruptured abdominal aortic aneurysm (AAA)

Diagnosis

Time is critical if you suspect a patient has a ruptured AAA. The patient should get to theatre without delay – call for senior help the moment you receive the GP call. The patient should be assessed in a high-dependency area, ideally theatre recovery. The key to treatment is early senior review close to theatre. Suspect the diagnosis in a patient with collapse or hypotension and a palpable or known aneurysm.

What to do

- If the patient is shocked:
  - call your senior immediately
  - give the patient O_2 via a non-rebreathing mask with 10 L flow
  - insert two large-bore cannulae in the antecubital fossae
  - take bloods for FBC, U+Es, coagulation studies and cross-match 6–8 units of blood
  - give colloid as quickly as possible through both cannulae to try and maintain the blood pressure above 80–90 systolic. Give blood as soon as it is available.
- As soon as senior help arrives, get the patient to theatre. The only thing that is going to help the patient with a ruptured AAA is surgical intervention.
- If the patient is not shocked:
  - take a very brief history: the patient might have a history of known AAA but can present with hypovolaemic shock and the clinical signs of a ruptured aneurysm – severe back pain, distended, tender abdomen, feeling faint. There might be a history of ischaemic heart disease.
- On examination: usually a tender abdomen with a palpable pulsatile mass. Monitor vital signs frequently.
- Investigations and management: if the patient is not shocked but you still think there is a ruptured aneurysm, then still call for senior help to help confirm the diagnosis and prepare the patient for theatre. Take blood as above. Imaging has no place unless there are serious doubts about the diagnosis.

Points to watch

- If you suspect the diagnosis, act quickly. Do not be put off by the fact that the patient seems stable at the present time; the next fall in blood pressure could be the last.
- A proportion of patients with a leaking or ruptured AAA will stand very little chance of surviving surgery; especially frail patients with coexisting heart and lung disease. Discuss these patients with your senior before suggesting that surgery is the correct option.

Acute pancreatitis

Diagnosis

Patients with pancreatitis need to be monitored very closely. They can deteriorate rapidly, with multiple organ systems affected. Consider the diagnosis on any patient with epigastric or back pain, persistent vomiting or a history of gallstones or alcoholism. Diagnosis is usually confirmed by an amylase of > 500 U/L; amylase can fall if presentation is late.

What to do

- Take a history. Patients present with severe central abdominal/epigastric pain, which can radiate to the back.

- Check for risk factors by thinking of the causes of pancreatitis:

Gall stones	**S**teroids and diabetes
Ethanol	**M**umps and other viral infections such as Coxsackie A
Trauma	**S**corpion bites
	Hyperlipidaemia and hypercalcaemia
	ERCP
	Drugs, e.g. azathioprine and thiazide diuretics.

- On examination: check for fever. Check pulse and BP for haemodynamic instability. Check for central/epigastric abdominal tenderness. Listen to the chest for signs of pleural and pericardial effusions; check the respiratory rate and O_2 saturations.

- Investigations: these are usually geared to give an indication of the severity of the attack and a guide to prognosis using scoring systems such as the modified Ranson criteria, which uses a combination of clinical and biochemical features to estimate severity:

  - FBC: check for anaemia and DIC; a raised WCC is common
  - U+Es: a raised creatinine is a poor prognostic indicator
  - LFTs: an obstructive picture with raised ALP and bilirubin and normal or mildly raised AST/ALT can give a clue to the underlying cause – gallstones might be present. Also ask for AST and LDH
  - amylase is a sensitive marker of pancreatitis but some units now use lipase
  - INR
  - glucose (raised in severe pancreatitis)
  - calcium (low in severe pancreatitis)
  - blood gases: a baseline pH, base excess and pO_2 on air gives essential information regarding the severity of the attack
  - chest X-ray: look for signs of a pleural effusion or adult respiratory distress syndrome
  - abdominal X-ray: calcification around the pancreas suggests chronic pancreatitis.

All units should now have a risk scoring proforma based on the Ranson criteria which will stratify the patient into mild, moderate and severe catagories. Make sure that these are utilized. They have trigger points which will identify the patient who requires early ITU review. Use and follow their recommendations.

Management

- Analgesia: 5–10 mg IV morphine stat and up to 4 hourly; 50 mg cyclizine IV/IM/PO. The patient might need a PCA pump – discuss this with your seniors.
- Oxygen: give the patient O_2 via non-rebreathing mask, even if the O_2 saturations are maintained.
- Fluids: a 1-L bag of IV normal saline should be given over 1 h, then over 2 h, 4 h and then 4–6-hourly thereafter. Insert a urethral catheter and monitor the urine output hourly. Increase fluids if this is not maintained between at least 30 and 60 mL an hour.
- 4-hourly BM measurements.
- Low-molecular-weight heparin and TEDs for DVT prophylaxis.
- Measure daily U+Es and amylase.
- Organize an urgent abdominal ultrasound of the pancreas and liver to look for gallstones or common bile duct dilation. If stones are seen, the patient might need an ERCP.

Points to watch

- If the patient is unwell and haemodynamically compromised, call for senior help. Patients with pancreatitis can deteriorate very rapidly; HDU/ITU help should be sought sooner rather than later; use your local proforma to risk stratify your patient.
- Keep an eye on O_2 saturations. Adult respiratory distress syndrome can occur; consult ITU sooner rather than later.
- Beware of raised glucose and treat with a sliding scale.
- Antibiotics are not routinely required for pancreatitis unless signs of infection are present elsewhere (e.g. chest, UTI) or dead pancreas is seen on CT scanning – consult your seniors.
- If bleeding occurs, check clotting, D-dimers and platelets for disseminated intravascular coagulation.

Bowel obstruction

Diagnosis

The hallmarks are colicky pain, nausea and vomiting, a distended, tender abdomen, with hyperactive bowel sounds. Diagnosis is usually confirmed on abdominal X-ray.

What to do

- Take a history: look for abdominal pain, nausea and vomiting. Has the patient ever had any abdominal surgery? Ask when the bowels last opened and when the patient last passed wind. Ask about previous symptoms such as weight loss and change in bowel habit.

- On examination, note vital signs and temperature. Check hernial orifices for strangulated/fixed hernias, look for visible peristalsis, feel the abdomen and listen for bowel sounds.

- Perform a rectal examination to search for any malignancy and degree of constipation.

- Any signs of peritonitis (guarding and rebound tenderness) suggest perforation or strangulation – both these require urgent surgical intervention. Get your senior to confirm the diagnosis and prepare the patient for theatre.

- Investigations: a cannula should be inserted and bloods taken for FBC, U+Es, glucose, amylase; cross-match 2 units. Do an erect chest X-ray to exclude perforation, plus a plain abdominal X-ray (erect or supine). Do a blood gas; worsening acidosis suggests dying bowel.

- Keep the patient nil by mouth.

- Give 1-L bags of IV normal saline over 1, 2, 4 and 6 h.

- Give 5–10 mg IV morphine stat and up to 4-hourly with 50 mg IV cyclizine.

- Insert an NG tube.

- Omit low-molecular-weight heparin prophylaxis in case surgery is required; use TEDs for DVT prophylaxis.

- If the patient is due for a laparotomy, cross-match 4 units of blood (check local policy) and consent patient for theatre.

Points to note

> ### Causes of Obstruction:
> **Small bowel:**
> - hernias • adhesions • Crohn's disease • intussusception
>
> **Large bowel:**
> - constipation • colonic carcinoma • diverticular stricture • sigmoid volvulus

Pseudo-obstruction – where no mechanical cause is found and an underlying biochemical, drug or medical cause (e.g. systemic infection) – causes gut paralysis. These patients have a cavernous rectum and can be relieved by a dupeza drain placed by a finger into the rectum.

- Further investigations: once the patient is stable, the cause of obstruction should be sought, e.g. large bowel obstruction should be investigated with double-contrast barium enema or colonoscopy.

Diverticulitis

Diagnosis

Think of the diagnosis in patients with left iliac fossa pain or tenderness. Diverticular disease can present with any number of symptoms ranging from abdominal pain and vomiting to perforation and shock. Localized inflammation of one or more diverticulae can cause localized peritonitis, which should be treated conservatively if possible, although surgical intervention will be required if it perforates or for repeated episodes.

What to do

- Check ABC. Patients are often elderly and do not tolerate systemic infection well.
- Check O_2 saturations and give O_2. Put in a large peripheral cannula and start IV fluids. If the systolic BP is less than 100 mmHg, give fast IV colloids and call your senior.
- Take a history: patients present with lower abdominal pain, commonly in the left iliac fossa. This can be associated with nausea and vomiting. There is often a history of constipation. Ask women about the possibility of pregnancy and pelvic infection. Ask about comorbid disease, especially cardiorespiratory disease.
- Check vital signs and temperature.
- Examine the abdomen for tenderness, guarding and rebound. If it is rigid with generalized tenderness, suspect perforation. Do a PR exam to check for bleeding, tumours and constipation.
- Take blood for FBC, U+Es, amylase, glucose, group and save.
- Check urine for protein/blood and do pregnancy test on women.
- If patient has a fever, send blood cultures.
- Perform an erect chest X-ray to exclude perforation.
- Give 5–10 mg IV morphine stat and up to 4-hourly with 50 mg IV cyclizine.
- Give normal saline IV 1-L bags 1-, 2-, 4- and 6-hourly.
- If patient has a fever, give IV cefuroxime 750 mg three times a day and IV metronidazole 500 mg three times a day.
- Give TEDs and low-molecular-weight heparin to prevent DVT.
- If the patient has perforated, group and save and consent for laparotomy.

Points to note

DIFFERENTIAL DIAGNOSIS
- Perforation of any other cause (especially sigmoid carcinoma).
- Colitis.
- In women:
    - ruptured ectopic pregnancy
    - pelvic inflammatory disease
    - tubal abscess
    - ovarian cyst (torsion).

- Many patients with diverticulitis settle on antibiotics. If the patient fails to settle, consider a diverticular abscess; get an urgent ultrasound scan to look for a collection.
- Diverticulitis can present with bleeding; also remember that fistulae can form between the bowel and the vagina or the bladder.
- Sigmoid cancer can present in an identical way to diverticular disease; follow-up examination with barium enema is necessary to exclude this.

Perforation

Diagnosis

About 70% of patients with a perforated viscus have air under the diaphragm on an erect chest X-ray. X-rays should be assessed in conjunction with the clinical signs – diffuse guarding and rebound tenderness in a very unwell patient point to the diagnosis. The crucial point in their symptoms is the rapidity of onset, 'it happened at ten past one', 'I was just bending down to open the fridge when', perforation is a sudden event.

What to do

- Start with ABC.
- Check for low O_2 saturations and give 100% O_2. Check pulse and BP; if BP is low, put in two large-bore peripheral cannulae and start a fast colloid infusion. Call your senior.
- Take a brief history: patients usually present with a short history of generalized abdominal pain made worse by movement or coughing. Take a full drug history including ulcer disease, alcohol and NSAID use. Note preceding symptoms such as weight loss, anorexia or change in bowel habit. Check for any significant past medical history.
- Check vital signs and temperature.
- Examine the abdomen for signs of peritonitis (tenderness, guarding, rebound). Check carefully for bowel sounds – if the patient has perforated these will usually be absent.
- Investigations: the diagnostic investigation is the erect chest X-ray; call for senior help immediately if there is air under the diaphragm. If the patient cannot tolerate sitting up, ask for a decubitus abdominal film (taken lying on the side). Take bloods for FBC, U+Es, glucose, LFTs, amylase. Group and save blood ready for laparotomy.
- Perform a plain abdominal X-ray.
- Keep the patient nil by mouth and consider NG tube.
- Give plenty of fluids – normal saline IV 1-L bags over 1, 2, 4 and 6 h.
- Give 5–10 mg IV morphine stat and up to 4 hourly with 50 mg IV cyclizine.
- Give antibiotics. IV cefuroxime 750 mg and IV metronidazole 500 mg.
- Consent the patient for a laparotomy.

> ### Common causes of perforation/generalized peritonitis:
> • Perforated peptic ulcer (gastric or duodenal) • Gastric carcinoma • Colonic carcinoma • Burst diverticulum • Perforated appendix

Points to watch

- Involve your seniors early – patients with perforation are very unwell and need speedy surgery (ideally within 6–8 h of onset). Mortality rises with time.
- Absence of air under the diaphragm on chest X-ray does not exclude the diagnosis.

Ischaemic gut

Diagnosis

A diagnosis of an ischaemic gut is usually made once all other diagnoses have been excluded. The diagnosis is suggested if the patient's symptoms are disproportionate to the abdominal signs – peritonism is a late finding. Shock is a common accompaniment to ischaemic gut.

What to do

- Start with ABC. The patient could be unwell from another cause, e.g. hypovolaemic, cardiogenic or septic shock, leading to poor gut blood supply.
- Put in at least one large cannula.
- Ensure the patient is well oxygenated (do not rely on O_2 saturations because the patient might be shut down peripherally) and, if hypotensive, give fast IV colloid.
- Take a brief history: the typical picture is a short history of abdominal pain, which is generalized and sometimes associated with nausea and vomiting. A past history of ischaemic heart disease or atrial fibrillation might be present but ischaemia may occur in the absence of these factors.
- On examination, check vital signs and temperature. There are usually very few signs to be found, although abdominal tenderness might be a feature. Examine the cardiovascular system, looking for atrial fibrillation, missing pulses, signs of endocarditis. Look for signs of stroke.
- Investigations:
  - routine bloods for FBC, U+Es, LFTs, CRP, glucose, amylase, group and save
  - arterial blood gases – look for a metabolic acidosis and for hypoxia
  - premenopausal women should have a pregnancy test
  - urine dipstick and MSU
  - ECG – look for AF or evidence of ischaemia
  - erect chest X-ray and abdominal X-ray.
- Give 100% O_2.
- IV normal saline should be given in 1-L bags over 4–6 h; give faster if the patient is shocked.
- Give 5–10 mg IV morphine stat and up to 4-hourly with 50 mg IV cyclizine.
- TED stockings and low-molecular-weight heparin to prevent DVT.
- Once a diagnosis has been made, the patient should undergo an urgent laparotomy and have the area of ischaemic gut resected.

Lower GI Bleed

Diagnosis

Fresh blood passed rectally. Ensure that the blood is coming from the rectum, rather than the urethra or vagina.

What to do

- Start with ABC.
- Ensure that at least one large peripheral cannula is in place. Take blood for FBC, U+Es, group and save. Check pulse and blood pressure; give fast IV colloid if pulse > 100 or systolic BP < 100.
- Take a history: fresh blood suggests a rectal or perianal bleed and is more common in younger patients. Partially altered blood and clots suggest colonic bleeding and tend to be found in older patients. Is there a history of anaemia? Ask about weight loss and a history of a change in bowel habit.
- Take a full drug history: is the patient on warfarin or NSAIDs? Ask about alcohol use.
- Check vital signs and look for signs of weight loss or bleeding elsewhere. Examine the abdomen for masses or enlarged liver or spleen. Perform a rectal examination and examine the perianal area for evidence of fresh blood.
- Take blood for FBC, U+Es, amylase, clotting screen, group and save.
- If the patient has fresh blood present, organize a flexible sigmoidoscopy once the bleeding has settled. If the patient has altered blood PR, organize either a barium enema or a colonoscopy once the bleeding has settled.
- Conservative management should be pursued if possible. If the patient is shocked, resuscitate with IV colloid through two large-bore cannulae and call for senior help. Group and save and transfuse if Hb < 9.
- If the patient is stable: give fluids – IV normal saline over 4–6 h. If the patient is anaemic and requires transfusion, give blood as necessary to raise the haemoglobin to 10 g/dL.

Points to note

Although alarming for the patient, lower GI bleeds tend to settle with conservative management. Patients who undergo acute surgical intervention usually undergo a total colectomy because the source of bleeding might not be isolated. This is best avoided unless unquenchable haemorrhage supervenes.

Differential diagnosis of lower GI bleeding

- Diverticulitis • Colorectal cancer/polyps • Haemorrhoids • Angiodysplasia
- Meckel's diverticulum

Strangulated hernia

Diagnosis

Diagnosis is on clinical grounds – a fixed, irreducible, tender lump in one of the hernial orifices. It might be associated with features of bowel obstruction or peritonitis.

What to do

- Start with a history: patients usually present with a known history of a hernia that becomes tender and fixed. They might also present with generalized abdominal pain and signs of obstruction.
- Examination: examine the hernia, looking for tenderness, reducibility, colour changes on the overlying skin and the presence of bowel sounds. Examine the abdomen for tenderness, distension and bowel sounds. Do not try too hard to reduce a tender hernia – you could merely exacerbate any soiling of the peritoneum if perforation has occurred.
- Investigations: take blood for FBC, U+Es, glucose, amylase, CRP, group and save. Perform an abdominal X-ray to exclude any signs of small or large bowel obstruction. Perform an erect chest X-ray to look for perforation.
- Keep the patient nil by mouth.
- Give 5–10 mg IV morphine stat and up to 4-hourly with 50 mg IV cyclizine.
- Give normal saline IV 1-L bags over 4–6 h. If signs of obstruction are present, give more frequently. If the patient is shocked, give fast IV colloid and call your senior immediately.
- If the patient has a tender fixed hernia, this should be repaired as soon as possible. Discuss with your seniors and consent the patient for surgery.

Points to watch

Strangulated hernia cannot be diagnosed unless you check the hernial orifices. Femoral hernias are especially likely to strangulate. Do not forget that hernias can occur around the umbilicus, in old scars and in the obturator canal as well as in the inguinal and femoral areas.

Biliary colic and cholecystitis

Diagnosis

Suspect in patients with right upper quadrant pain. The presence of guarding, rebound tenderness, leucocytosis and fever are pointers to acute cholecystitis.

What to do

- Take a history: patients present with right upper quadrant pain, which is usually colicky in nature. It is associated with nausea and might have occurred previously on eating fatty foods. Check previous history of gallstones; also ask about alcohol consumption, ulcer disease and risk factors for previous pancreatitis. Are there any risk factors for hepatitis as an alternative diagnosis?

- Examination: check vital signs and temperature. Examine for signs of jaundice and hepatomegaly. Examine the abdomen for right upper quadrant tenderness and guarding. Look for Murphy's sign (pain in inspiration when palpating the right upper quadrant). Listen to the lungs for signs of a right basal pneumonia which can mimic cholecystitis.

- Investigations:
  - take blood for FBC, CRP, U+Es, glucose, LFTs, amylase, INR, group and save
  - do an erect chest X-ray and plain abdominal X-ray
  - if the patient has a fever, take blood cultures
  - send an MSU.

- Keep patient nil by mouth.
- Give 5–10 mg IV morphine stat and up to 4-hourly with 50 mg IV cyclizine.
- Give IV normal saline 1-L bags 2-hourly, 4-hourly then 6-hourly.
- Check FBC and CRP daily.
- If patient has a fever or a high WCC, treat as acute cholecystitis. Treat with IV cefuroxime 750 mg three times a day and IV metronidazole 500 mg three times a day, or IV ciprofloxacin (check your local policy).
- Organize abdominal ultrasound to confirm the diagnosis and look for gallstones. A dilated common bile duct might require further investigation with ERCP.

Points to watch

Cholecystectomy can be performed early (< 48 hours) or late (> 6 weeks) in a reasonably straightforward manner. In between these times the decision is more difficult.

- If patient has jaundice, fever and abdominal pain, treat for ascending cholangitis with IV cefuroxime and metronidazole, or IV ciprofloxacin. Consider IV gentamicin in cases of severe sepsis. Get an urgent abdominal ultrasound; a blocked infected bile duct might need ERCP to remove any stones, otherwise the infection is unlikely to resolve.

Acute limb ischaemia

Diagnosis

Is on clinical grounds – rapid onset of a painful, pulseless, paraesthetic, paralysed, perishingly cold limb. The diagnosis is confirmed by Doppler studies and angiography.

What to do

- Take a brief history: sudden onset pain and numbness in a limb is typical. Ask about previous episodes and any episode of loss of motor function. Any neurological deficit is a surgical emergency because the artery must be reopened within 6 h to prevent permanent damage. Check for a previous history of AF, recent MI (mural thrombus), IHD or PVD, and previous aortic or mitral valve disease.
- Examination: examine the limb thoroughly. It is usually mottled and dusky with poor/absent peripheral pulses and reduced sensation. Check motor function. Examine the heart and peripheral pulses. Check for an AAA.
- Send bloods for FBC, U+Es, glucose, clotting screen. Perform an ECG looking for atrial fibrillation or recent myocardial infarction.
- Give O_2.
- Give 5–10 mg IV morphine stat and up to 4-hourly with 50 mg IV cyclizine.
- Anticoagulate: give IV heparin 5000 U stat followed by an infusion of 24 000 U over 24 h. Check APTTr every 6 h and maintain at 2–3. Low molecular weight heparin is used by some units as an alternative.
- Treatment is complex. This will need to be discussed with your seniors in conjunction with the radiologists.
- Surgery (embolectomy) is not usually considered unless the patient is known to have had relatively normal arteries previously with no history of intermittent claudication, there is an obvious source for the clot (e.g. a mural thrombus postmyocardial infarction), and that contralateral pulses are all normal.

Points to watch

- Time is of the essence. Tell your senior at an early stage so that the appropriate investigations and interventions can be arranged within 6 h of symptom onset.
- Reperfusion problems include release of potassium and myoglobin from damaged tissue. Keep a close eye on potassium postoperatively and check the creatine kinase. Ensure that the patient stays well hydrated and aim for a urine output of > 100 mL/h to flush myoglobin through and prevent acute renal failure.
- Late presentations might not be salvageable; amputation might be the only feasible option.

Testicular torsion

Diagnosis

Suspect testicular torsion on any patient with rapid onset of testicular pain, especially if unilateral. Do not assume that the condition is due to epididymo-orchitis.

What to do

- Take a history: torsion usually affects males under the age of 30. The typical presentation is with rapid onset pain (< 30 min) and nausea. Ask if this has happened before. Is there a history of mumps, sore throat, penile discharge or pain passing urine? Is there a history of trauma to the scrotum?

- Examination is not usually tolerated but the affected testis rides higher than the unaffected side and there can be associated right iliac fossa tenderness and loin pain.

- Inform your senior at an early stage that a possible torsion case is in the hospital – this condition should be treated as urgently as a ruptured aneurysm.

- Take routine bloods including WCC and CRP – these are usually normal.

- Check urine dipstick – this is usually also normal.

- Get an urgent testicular ultrasound once adequate analgesia has been given; this is the best non-invasive test to distinguish from epidymo-orchitis.

- Give 5–10 mg IV morphine stat and up to 4-hourly with 50 mg IV cyclizine. Diclofenac 75–100 mg PR is an alternative.

- If the patient has a torsion, the treatment is surgical and the patient should be consented for an orchidopexy, where both testes are tied to the scrotal sac. If there is any evidence of infarction at operation, the testis is removed. This should be clearly stated to the patient and documented.

Points to note

Epidymo-orchitis – inflammation of the testes – usually presents in older men and is bilateral. There is also an associated history of infection, such as rigors with fever. The urine dipstick is positive for protein and there is an elevated WCC and raised inflammatory markers. The treatment is bed-rest and antibiotics (such as ciprofloxacin). Mumps should be considered in young men.

If there is any doubt as to the diagnosis, and testicular ultrasound is delayed, exploratory surgery should proceed without delay. Torsion of the testis results in infarction and death of the testicle in 6–8 h.

Acute urinary retention

Diagnosis

Patients present unable to pass urine with an enlarged painful bladder. The diagnosis is on clinical grounds, confirmed by passing a urinary catheter.

What to do

- Examine the patient to confirm the presence of a bladder, then pass a urethral catheter to relieve the symptoms. Take a full history later – the patient will never be more grateful!

- Take a history: in men, the most common cause of urinary retention is prostate enlargement. Ask about obstructive features such as nocturia, frequency, poor stream, hesitancy and postmicturition dribbling. Also ask about dysuria, haematuria and abdominal pain. In both men and women, urinary infections and constipation can also cause retention. Bear in mind neurological causes of retention such as spinal cord compression.

- Examination: once you have examined the patient's abdomen and diagnosed and treated the acute retention, perform a rectal examination to look for faecal loading and to assess prostate size.

- Investigations: check FBC and U+Es. Check CRP if you suspect infection. PSA might not be helpful at this stage because it might be elevated by infection, rectal examination and the passage of the catheter.

- Send a catheter urine specimen for microscopy and culture.

Points to watch

- Measurement of the residual bladder volume is crucial – a large volume (> 1 L) suggests poor bladder compliance due to chronic partial obstruction.

- If the U+Es suggest acute renal failure, the patient needs an urgent renal ultrasound to exclude obstruction and hydronephrosis (see 'Acute renal failure', p. 117, for further details).

- All patients should be admitted and their urine output monitored. They might develop polyuria when their obstruction is removed, in which case they will need IV fluid replacement to prevent dehydration. Use the amount of urine passed in the previous hour plus 30 mL as a guide as to how much fluid (normal saline) to give per hour if the patient is polyuric.

- Once the patient is stable, the underlying problem should be treated, e.g. constipation or UTI. Men with enlarged prostates can be discharged and brought back to hospital for a trial without catheter. Further management can then be decided (e.g. alpha-blockers or surgery with TURP).

- Painless retention, especially with a lax anal sphincter, suggests cord compression or cauda equina compression. Discuss with your seniors urgently regarding spinal cord imaging.

Renal colic

Diagnosis

Suspect the diagnosis in patients with waves of flank pain, usually accompanied by nausea and vomiting.

What to do

- Take a brief history: patients present with unilateral loin pain, which is severe and radiates down to the groin (or testes in men) with associated nausea. There might be a previous history of stone disease.
- Examination: patients with renal colic are frequently doubled up in pain. Give analgesia quickly. Check vital signs and temperature. Examine the abdomen for flank tenderness and fullness (infection or obstruction). Perform a rectal examination in men to assess prostate size if bilateral obstruction is suspected. Always examine peripheral pulses and exclude an abdominal artery aneurysm.
- Take blood for FBC, WCC, U+Es, amylase. Check urine for blood on disptick and send an MSU.
- Perform a KUB X-ray to look for evidence of stones. Follow along the tips of the transverse processes to the pelvis and then along the sacroiliac joints to trace the ureters. Check the renal shadows for signs of enlargement.
- If patient has a fever, send blood cultures.
- Patients will need an IVU (intravenous urogram) or more commonly a CT of the kidney, ureters and bladder (CT-KUB) to look for stones or any obstruction. This can be done the next day unless there is any suggestion of infection or obstruction. In this situation the diagnosis needs to be made and the obstruction relieved otherwise the kidney will be permanently damaged.
- Give diclofenac PR 75–100 mg 12–18-hourly; opiates can also be useful.
- Give IV normal saline 4–6-hourly to help flush the kidneys and pass the stone.
- Most stones will pass down the ureter and out in the urine with time. If it is large, lithotripsy can be used to fracture it into smaller pieces. If there is a significant obstruction, a percutaneous nephrostomy will need to be performed.

Points to note

- Aortic aneurysm: left-sided renal colic in older men should raise the suspicion of a leaking abdominal aortic aneurysm. Talk to your senior urgently if you can feel an AAA.
- Other differential diagnoses include: ureteric stricture, TCC of ureter, sloughed renal papillae and pelvic–ureteric junction obstruction.
- If the patient has a fever or is in acute renal failure, get an urgent ultrasound to ascertain whether the kidney is completely obstructed. Kidneys that are infected or obstructed by ureteric stones need urgent decompression, usually with a nephrostomy tube placed under radiological guidance.

Medical presentations

The sick patient

It does not require a medical degree to recognize a sick patient; it is usually fairly obvious. Sadly, this ability is sometimes lost during medical training, leading to delay in treatment and potentially to lost lives. Trusts are increasingly using scoring systmes (eg Patient At Risk (PAR) score) in order to help identify the sickest patients.

When assessing a patient, always start with ABC:

- Airway
- Breathing
- Circulation

Although often quoted, this rule is crucial in patient management. Quite often you will make this judgement in a split-second – the patient is sitting up in bed, talking and in no obvious distress – but remember to use it in all situations as a framework.

Linked with ABC are vital signs. They are called vital signs for a very good reason. Blood pressure, pulse and respiratory rate are always important in patient assessment.

Airway

Assessing airway patency Signs of complete obstruction include absent breath sounds, paradoxical ('seesaw') breathing and eventually cyanosis. Partial obstruction is accompanied by stridor – do not confuse stridor with wheeze; wheeze is expiratory, stridor is inspiratory.

Management If there is any sign of airways obstruction, call for senior help – the patient will need the obstruction removed and might need ventilating. Consider inserting a Guedel airway or a nasopharyngeal airway. Don't go on to B and C until you have secured the airway.

Breathing

If the patient is breathless, check the respiratory rate, O_2 saturations and arterial blood gases. Examine the chest looking for signs of a pneumothorax (check for mediastinal shift and a tension pneumothorax if the patient is hypotensive), pneumonia, left ventricular failure or COPD/asthma. Hyperventilation is often diagnosed by more senior members of staff – take a blood gas and make sure the patient is not hyperventilating appropriately, e.g. if hypoxic or from a metabolic acidosis. Be very cautious about diagnosing hyperventilation due to anxiety; the patient might die if you are wrong.

Management Treat a hypoxic patient with O_2. Be cautious in patients with COPD because they need controlled O_2 therapy with regular monitoring of their CO_2. Remember, however, that patients with COPD die from hypoxia – not from hypercapnia. If the pO_2 is < 8 kPa on arterial blood gases, use a non-rebreathing mask with the reservoir filled with O_2. Ensure the O_2 flow rate is 10 L/min and that the reservoir does not collapse with inspiration. If the patient is still hypoxic, call for senior help. Many more people die of hypoxia than die of inappropriately vigorous O_2 therapy. Look for the cause, i.e. clinical examination and chest X-ray, and begin treating appropriately.

Circulation

The most common vital sign to be recorded is blood pressure; when this drops, the patient has lost a lot of circulating volume. Tachycardia is an earlier sign of haemodynamic compromise and so should be taken seriously, e.g. in hypovolaemic shock. Capillary refill time (usually < 2 s) can also be helpful as an end-of-the-bed test for circulatory compromise.

Management If the patient is tachycardic, i.e. pulse > 100, with a normal blood pressure, perform an ECG to exclude arrhythmias. If the patient is in sinus rhythm there might be an underlying cause. These include bleeding, dehydration, infection, pulmonary embolism. Fluid resuscitation with IV colloid (given through a wide-bore peripheral cannula) should be given if hypovolaemia is suspected.

If the patient is hypotensive, establish the cause, i.e. hypovolaemic, cardiogenic, anaphylactic or septic shock. All but cardiogenic shock require IV fluid resuscitation.

Conscious level

The Glasgow Coma Scale (GCS) is universally used to describe conscious state. It is scored by assessing the patient's best eye response, verbal response and movement responses. It is scored out of 15, the minimum being 3. Any patient with a GCS of < 14 should be discussed with your senior. Any drop in GCS of two or more points should also raise alarm bells. Any patient with a GCS < 9 should be considered for ventilation because they might have lost airway protective reflexes.

The GCS makes up part of the neurological observations that can be performed on the wards. These should be done on patients with suspected cranial pathology, e.g. head injuries, stroke or intracranial haemorrhage.

Glasgow coma scale:

Eyes

4	Spontaneous eye opening
3	Eyes open to voice or command
2	Eyes open to painful stimulus – usually to limb or trunk
1	Eyes remain closed

Voice

5	Orientated speech
4	Confused speech
3	Inappropriate speech – occasional words but not coherent
2	Incomprehensible speech – groans and muttering
1	No speech

Motor response

6	Obeys commands
5	Localizes to pain – uses limb to localize or fight
4	Withdrawal to painful stimulus
3	Abnormal flexor response
2	Extensor response to painful stimulus
1	No response to painful stimuli

Score each section individually, then give the total, e.g. E = 3; M = 4; V = 4; Total = 11/15

Chest pain

Assess patients with chest pain quickly. Look at their vital signs and the ECG as soon as they arrive. If they are in respiratory distress, see 'Shortness of breath' (p. 156); if they are hypotensive, see 'Shock' (p. 158). Obtain IV access early in case of cardiac arrest.

History

Take a brief history. Note the onset of pain (gradual in ischaemic pain and pneumonia) or sudden (PE, pneumothorax, aortic dissection):

- Is the pain dull and retrosternal, or pleuritic?
- When did it start? This is particularly important when considering thrombolysis.
- What makes it better or worse? (e.g. GTN, inspiration).
- Ask about associated features, e.g. nausea, vomiting, sweating, cough, haemoptysis.
- Note any risk factors for thromboembolic or cardiac disease, and note any previous history of angina, MI other cardiorespiratory disease.

Examination

- Do the pulse, blood pressure in each arm, respiratory rate and O_2 saturations.
- Thoroughly examine the heart and lungs – are there signs of consolidation or any tenderness on pressing the chest wall?
- Do a peak flow if you suspect asthma.
- Check for leg swelling – CCF or DVT.

Investigations

- FBC, U+Es, glucose, CRP.
- 12 hour troponin.
- Arterial blood gases: if $SaO_2 < 95\%$ or if the patient is tachypnoeic.
- ECG: look for evidence of MI or acute coronary syndrome (see 'ECG abnormalities', p. 215); arrhythmias including AF and sinus tachycardia (due to infection or PE).
- Chest X-ray: signs of consolidation, pneumothorax, wide mediastinum, LVF or effusion.

Management

- Resuscitate the patient if necessary – ABC.
- Establish a diagnosis – treat the cause.
- If you think that the pain is cardiac in origin give:
  - O_2 (100%)
  - analgesia: 2.5–5 mg diamorphine IV or morphine 5–10 mg IV; 10 mg metoclopromide IV
  - 300 mg aspirin unless contraindicated.

- If ST elevation or new left bundle branch block: contact your senior immediately to discuss thrombolysis.
- If there is ST depression or deep T wave inversion give 300 mg Clopidogrel PO in addition to aspirin.
- Otherwise, anticoagulate with heparin (unfractionated or LMWH) and start a GTN infusion/sublingual nitrates if still in pain.
- If you think that the pain is respiratory give:
  - O_2 (100% unless known COPD)
  - adequate analgesia – oral if possible; diamorphine in extreme situations (respiratory depressant).
- Treat the cause – anticoagulate if PE, antibiotics if fever or consolidation, aspiration or chest drain if pneumothorax on chest X-ray; diuretics for pulmonary oedema.

Other diagnoses to consider

- Peptic ulcer disease/gastro-oesophageal reflux.
- Pericarditis (saddle-shaped ST segments on ECG).
- Aortic dissection (unequal blood pressures, wide mediastinum on chest X-ray, tearing pain to the back). Call your senior immediately.
- Cholecystitis, pancreatitis.
- Musculoskeletal chest pain (look for tenderness over chest wall that reproduces pain).
- Oesophageal rupture (the patient is usually very unwell; look for mediastinal gas on chest X-ray).

Acute breathlessness

Resuscitation

- Your initial assessment should include:
  - A: assessment of airway to exclude obstruction
  - B: note of vital signs, i.e. respiratory rate, O_2 saturations and arterial blood gases
  - C: pulse and blood pressure.
- If the patient is cyanotic with very slow breathing, put out an arrest call.
- If the patient is hypoxic, treat with O_2 after taking a blood gas sample.
- Make a rapid thorough examination of the patient's heart and lungs.

History

- Onset of breathlessness – sudden or gradual.
- Previous history of lung or heart disease, e.g. known heart failure or COPD.
- Associated symptoms, e.g. chest pain, haemoptysis, cough, temperature.
- Ask about the patient's usual exercise tolerance and smoking history.
- Make a list of important risk factors if you suspect PE or a cardiac cause.

Examination

- Vital signs – respiratory rate, O_2 saturations, BP, pulse, temperature.
- Look for signs of cyanosis and use of accessory muscles.
- Check JVP.
- Examine chest looking for signs of consolidation, LVF, pneumothorax or effusions.
- Examine the heart for gallop rhythm.
- Check legs for ankle oedema.

Investigations

- FBC, U+Es, glucose.
- 12 hour troponin.
- Arterial blood gases.
- ECG.
- Chest X-ray.
- Peak flow if the patient is known to be asthmatic.
- Sputum culture.

Diagnosis

The key to the diagnosis of acute breathlessness is the onset of symptoms.

If possible, wait for the chest X-ray before initiating treatment; if the patient is very unwell (e.g. acute pulmonary oedema), you will have to start treatment before radiographic confirmation of your diagnosis.

Diagnosis of acute breathlessness:

Sudden-onset breathlessness:

• pulmonary embolism • pneumothorax • pulmonary oedema

Gradual-onset breathlessness:

• pneumonia • exacerbation of asthma/COPD • pulmonary oedema

Management

- Correct hypoxia, using a non-rebreathing mask if necessary. Use caution if the patient has known or suspected COPD.

- Check ECG. Look for evidence of acute MI or arrhythmia and treat appropriately.

- Once you have made a provisional diagnosis, see the relevant chapters for treatment advice. Do not forget that more than one diagnosis could be coexisting, especially in older people.

- Regular monitoring of the patient's respiratory rate, O_2 saturations (and peak flow if necessary) is important. Remember that O_2 saturations should only be used as a guide – they can be dependent on a number of factors, e.g. contact with the patient's finger, peripheral circulation, presence of nail varnish.

Other diagnoses to consider

- Massive pleural effusion.

- Acute abdomen (pain and abdominal splinting cause breathlessness).

- Metabolic acidosis with compensatory hyperventilation, e.g. DKA, liver/renal failure, aspirin/paracetamol/tricyclic antidepressant overdose.

- Pancreatitis (causes metabolic acidosis and adult respiratory distress syndrome).

- Perforated oesophagus.

Hypotension

Patients with low blood pressure are usually very sick. Although they occasionally look well, they must be treated quickly before they decompensate. If you are asked to review someone with a low blood pressure (< 90 mmHg systolic), you must make this a priority. Anyone with a blood pressure of < 75 mmHg is very ill, particularly if they are peripherally shut down, oliguric or acidotic. They should be treated immediately. Call your senior.

History

Quite often, only a very brief history is available and treatment is begun simultaneously. Ask:

- What is their normal blood pressure? Some older people run a low blood pressure all the time, as do some young women. Interpret the blood pressure in the light of previous readings; a 'normal' blood pressure might be inappropriately low in someone who is hypertensive.
- Is there a history of infection, allergic reaction or a cardiac event?
- Is there a history of trauma, surgery or evidence of gastrointestinal bleeding?
- Does the patient have chest pain, abdominal pain, breathlessness, cough, urinary symptoms?
- Is the illness sudden in onset – think of massive PE, tension pneumothorax or a major cardiac event.
- Has the patient taken any medications that could lower blood pressure, e.g. ACE inhibitors, nitrates, beta-blockers.

Examination

- Look at the patient – Is the patient cold, clammy, sweaty warm or feverish? Check capillary return and assess their level of consciousness.
- Check the blood pressure yourself with a manual BP cuff.
- Examine for tracheal deviation to exclude tension pneumothorax.
- Examine the heart for murmurs, e.g. VSD, mitral regurgitation.
- Examine the chest for signs of poor air entry, pulmonary oedema or pneumothorax.
- Examine the abdomen for tenderness/masses. If the patient is stable, perform a PR examination looking for melaena or lower GI bleeding.

Investigations

- Insert two large-bore cannulae and take blood for FBC, U+Es, glucose and LFTs.
- Clotting screen and cross-match 6 units of blood if you suspect bleeding.
- ECG if you suspect cardiogenic shock; serum troponin at presentation and at 12 hours if the first negative.
- Blood cultures if sepsis is suspected (pyrexia or a temperature < 36 °C).
- ECG and Chest X-ray.

Diagnosis

- Cool peripheries, no JVP visible: hypovolaemia (e.g. bleeding, dehydration, some drugs), septic shock.
- Cool peripheries, JVP elevated: cardiogenic (e.g. MI, PE, tamponade, VSD or valve rupture, bradyarrhythmis or tachyarrhythmias).
- Warm peripheries, rash or wheeze: anaphylaxis.
- Warm peripheries, pyrexia: the patient is septic.

Management

- Give O_2 via a non-rebreathing mask.
- Insert a urinary catheter and monitor hourly urine output. Minimum urine output should be 30–40 mL/h (0.5 mL/kg/h).
- Further management is dependent on the underlying causes and should be undertaken with senior supervision:

Cardiogenic shock

- Transfer to CCU.
- Treat any underlying arrhythmia, e.g. ventricular tachycardia, complete heart block.
- If ST elevation or new left bundle branch block is present on ECG, thrombolyse with tPA or a derivative (avoid streptokinase because this could cause a further fall in blood pressure). Discuss with your registrar whether the patients should be considered for primary angioplasty at a specialist centre.
- An echo should be performed to look at LV function and to exclude cardiac tamponade, a VSD and any acute valve lesion.
- Ensure the patient is hydrated – a central line might need to be inserted but do not give fluid without consulting your senior.
- Give inotropic support, e.g. dobutamine 5–40 µg/kg/min.
- Management of massive pulmonary embolism is dealt with on p. 123.

Sepsis/anaphylaxis/hypovolaemia

- Adequate fluid resuscitation is crucial in these patients. Give IV colloid via large peripheral veins.
- If you suspect bleeding (look for GI bleeding, PV bleeding or PU bleeding), give blood as soon as you can.
- In sepsis, treat with appropriate IV antibiotics. If empirical treatment is required, a cephalosporin gives good all-round cover, e.g. IV cefuroxime 1.5 g 8-hourly.
- For anaphylaxis, give steroids, antihistamines and adrenaline if necessary.

Points to note

RARER CAUSES OF SHOCK

- Acute adrenal insufficiency. If a patient with a history of Addison's disease, hypopituitarism or long-term steroid use is hypotensive, give IV hydrocortisone 200 mg 6-hourly to cover adrenal insufficiency.
- Tension pneumothorax (see 'Pneumothorax', p. 129).

Hypertension

Patients presenting with uncontrolled hypertension are unusual and should be treated cautiously. Aggressive reduction in blood pressure can cause permanent neurological deficit. An underlying cause should also be sought, particularly if the patient is young.

History and examination

- Check the blood pressure yourself with a manual sphygmomanometer – do not trust electronic measurements. Check BP in both arms; take the higher reading. If systolic BP > 220 mmHg or diastolic > 130 mmHg, call your senior.
- Find out what the blood pressure usually runs at – this might not be a new finding at all. What other cardiovascular risk factors does the patient have?
- Look for evidence of hypertensive encephalopathy – headache, nausea, vomiting, confusion, fits, focal neurology, coma. Remember subarachnoid haemorrhage or stroke as your differential diagnoses; both events will cause hypertension. Discuss this with your senior for consideration of a CT head.
- Examine for evidence of hypertensive retinopathy – papilloedema, exudates or haemorrhages.
- Check urine for evidence of blood/protein.
- Send urgent U+Es to exclude acute renal failure.

Investigations

- FBC, U+Es, glucose, TFT.
- ECG.
- Chest X-ray.
- Consider CT head to exclude stroke, subarachnoid haemorrhage or other intracranial pathology.

Diagnoses

- Non-compliance with medication.
- Acute aortic dissection – check BP in both arms and peripheral pulses.
- Intracranial event – subarachnoid or intracerebral bleed, ischaemic stroke.
- Acute renal failure – glomerulonephritis.
- Renal artery stenosis.
- Phaeochromocytoma.
- Conn's syndrome.
- Cushing's syndrome.
- Drug abuse, e.g. amphetamines, cocaine.
- Anxiety.
- Pain.
- Many patients with uncontrolled hypertension will have 'primary' hypertension, i.e. no underlying cause will be found.

Management

Always discuss treatment with your senior – rapid reduction of blood pressure can be dangerous and cause stroke. There are very few occasions in which IV treatment is required.

- Start by ensuring that pain and anxiety are treated. If there are no signs of aortic dissection, encephalopathy or pulmonary oedema, there is no need to reduce the BP quickly. Watch and wait until the morning, or consider one of the following therapies:
  - amlodipine 5 mg once a day orally is good treatment in most situations
  - metoprolol 25 mg three times a day orally
  - bendroflumethazide 2.5 mg once daily
  - Note: avoid using sublingual nifedipine; this can cause sudden falls in blood pressure with the risk of watershed stroke.
- Intravenous therapy should always be reviewed by your senior and consideration should be given to an ITU admission with intra-arterial BP monitoring. Do not use intravenous therapy unless you suspect hypertensive encephalopathy, aortic dissection or hypertensive pulmonary oedema – sudden drops in blood pressure can cause stroke.
- GTN: 50 mg of GTN in 50 mL of normal saline starting at 2 mL/h.
- Labetalol: use if you suspect aortic dissection. Give 200 mg labetolol in 200 mL normal saline infused at 0.25 mg/min, increasing by 0.25 mg every 15–30 min with regular BP checks. Maximum dose 2 mg/min.

Tachycardias

Initial assessment with a patient with an uncontrolled tachycardia (HR > 120 bpm) must always include a 12-lead ECG to ascertain the rhythm, and a blood pressure measurement.

Resuscitation

Start with ABC. If the patient is hypotensive (systolic BP < 90 mmHg), call your senior immediately. In all but sinus tachycardia, any other adverse sign, e.g. reduced level of consciousness, pulmonary oedema or chest pain, should be treated with DC cardioversion.

History

- Ask about symptoms of chest pain, palpitations and breathlessness. If the patient has chest pain or breathlessness, try and time the onset of these symptoms with the palpitations.
- Any previous episodes? Any previous history of cardiac or thromboembolic disease?
- Full drug history, including recreational drug use. Include a smoking, caffeine and alcohol history.

Examination

- Vital signs and conscious level.
- Look for elevated JVP.
- Examine the heart for gallop and valve lesion.
- Examine the lungs for infection or pulmonary oedema.
- Examine the legs for swelling – DVT or peripheral oedema.

Investigations

- 12-lead ECG to examine rhythm and look for MI/ischaemia.
- FBC, U+Es, glucose, Mg^{2+}, Ca^{2+}, TFTs.
- 12-hour serum troponin.
- Chest X-ray.
- Arterial blood gas if the O_2 saturations are low or if you suspect pulmonary embolism.

Diagnosis

Diagnosis is based on the ECG. Tachycardia can be narrow complex (QRS < 0.12 s) or broad complex (QRS > 0.12 s).

SINUS TACHYCARDIA
- Usually a narrow complex, regular rhythm with a rate of 120 bpm or more.
- Often associated with underlying pathology – hypovolaemia, infection, PE.

ATRIAL FLUTTER
- Usually a narrow complex, regular rhythm, a rate of approximately 150 bpm suggests atrial flutter with 2:1 block.
- Can be associated with infections or PE, but can also be a primary cardiac problem.

ATRIAL FIBRILLATION
- Usually a narrow complex, irregular rhythm, rate up to 200 bpm.
- Like atrial flutter, atrial fibrillation can be due to underlying pathology or a primary cardiac cause.

SUPRAVENTRICULAR TACHYCARDIA
- Usually a narrow complex, regular rhythm, rate up to 250 bpm.
- Usually idiopathic but can be due to electrolyte disturbances, caffeine or drug ingestion, infections or PE.

VENTRICULAR TACHYCARDIA
- Broad complex, regular rhythm, rate up to 300 bpm.
- Always pathological. Underlying ischaemic heart disease must be excluded but can be due to drugs, particularly those that prolong QT interval, e.g. amiodarone, phenothiazines, tricyclic antidepressants or electrolyte imbalance.

Management
- Put the patient on a cardiac monitor.
- Give the patient O_2.
- Correct any electrolyte abnormalities (especially potassium and magnesium).
- Treat the underlying problem, e.g. infection, PE.
- If it is a primary arrhythmia, identify correctly (see 'ECG abnormalities', p. 215) and treat appropriately.

Bradycardias

Resuscitation

Start with ABC. If the heart rate is less than 60/min, assess the rhythm with 12-lead ECG and check the patient's blood pressure. If the BP is low, call your senior immediately and administer atropine 0.5–1 mg IV. Repeat up to a maximum of 3 mg. If there is no improvement, the patient should have a temporary pacing wire inserted with external pacing performed in the meantime.

History

- Any history of falls, dizziness, syncope or near syncope.
- Previous history of ischaemic heart disease.
- Full drug history, including eye-drops (beta-blocking eye-drops for glaucoma can cause bradycardia) and recreational drug use.
- Smoking and alcohol history.

Examination

- Vital signs and conscious level.
- JVP for presence of cannon waves (seen in complete heart block).
- Examine the heart for valve lesions.
- Examine the lungs for signs of pulmonary oedema.
- Examine the legs for ankle oedema.

Investigations

- 12-lead ECG to examine rhythm and look for acute MI/ischaemia.
- FBC, U+Es, glucose, Mg^{2+}, Ca^{2+}, TFT.
- 12 hour troponin
- Digoxin level (if appropriate).
- Chest X-ray.

Diagnosis

Sinus bradycardia Normal PR interval, i.e. from the beginning of the P wave to the beginning of R wave. QRS interval follows each P wave.

Junctional bradycardia Absent or inverted P waves or P waves following closely after the QRS complex.

1st degree AV block Prolonged PR interval (> 200 ms; five small squares) but each QRS preceded by a P wave.

2nd degree AV block Mobitz type 1 Gradual increase in PR interval followed by dropped beat. Also known as the Wenckebach phenomenon.

2nd degree AV block Mobitz type II Normal PR interval with occasional dropped beats; may be in a 2:1, 3:1 ratio.

3rd degree (complete) AV block No association between P wave and QRS complex.

Regular P waves (rate up to 150) and regular QRS complexes (rate around 40/min). QRS complexes are often broad.

Causes of bradycardia

• Drug overdose, e.g. beta-blockers, calcium channel antagonists

• Antiarrhythmic drugs • Digoxin toxicity • Underlying ischaemia, e.g. recent MI, (especially inferior MI) or acute coronary syndrome • Electrolyte imbalance, e.g. hyperkalaemia • Hypothermia, hypothyroidism

Many cases of heart block, especially in older people, are due to fibrosis of the conducting system. Occasionally, diseases such as endocarditis, rheumatic fever or sarcoidosis can cause heart block.

Management

- Put the patient on a cardiac monitor.

- Give the patient O_2.

- Correct any electrolyte abnormalities.

- Give atropine 600 µg IV up to a maximum of 3 mg; if there is no response and patient is compromised, call your senior because the patient might need a temporary pacing wire.

- If digoxin toxicity is suspected then correct any electrolyte abnormality (digoxin toxicity is more common in hypokalaemia, hypomagnesaemia and hypercalcaemia) and discuss with your senior regarding the use of Digibind antibodies.

- If beta-blocker overdose is suspected and there is no response to atropine, discuss with your senior and give IV glucagon 50 µg/kg as a bolus followed by an infusion of 1–5 mg/h.

- If drug treatment fails while waiting for a temporary wire, start external pacing from defibrillator. Sedation will usually be needed if the patient is conscious.

Nausea and vomiting

Very commonly seen on the wards as well as in patients presenting acutely on-take, particularly the elderly. Remember, nausea or vomiting might be the only symptom of a systemic infection or acute abdomen.

History

- Are the symptoms related to food? To medication?
- Ask about other symptoms, such as headache, abdominal pain, haematemesis, diarrhoea, constipation.
- Any other systemic features: sweating, fever, chest pain.
- Past medical history: Crohn's disease, diabetes, previous bowel surgery.
- Drug history: overdose, normal medication, recreational drug use.
- Alcohol history.

Examination

- Vital signs: pulse, BP, temperature.
- Skin: rashes or evidence of cellulitis.
- Abdominal examination: check for tenderness, distension and the presence of bowel sounds.
- Chest examination: murmurs or evidence of infection.
- Check for conscious level and neck stiffness. Is there papilloedema or photophobia?

Investigations

- FBC, U+Es, glucose, LFTs and calcium.
- Amylase.
- CRP.
- Erect chest X-ray and abdominal X-ray – look for perforation or bowel obstruction.

Differential diagnosis

- Gastroenteritis – usually viral.
- Drug reaction or overdose, including cytotoxic chemotherapy.
- Alcohol excess.
- Abdominal pathology: cholecystitis, pancreatitis.
- Bowel obstruction, constipation.
- Crohn's disease, peptic ulcer disease, gastritis, ureteric colic.
- Electrolyte imbalance, e.g. hypercalcaemia.
- Nausea/vomiting might be the only symptom of infection anywhere in an elderly patient.
- Pain and/or anxiety.

- Other diagnoses to bear in mind include DKA, MI and any other cause of an acute abdomen, e.g. appendicitis. In young women, don't forget pregnancy.

Management

- Rehydrate the patient: give IV fluids, usually normal saline.
- Correct any electrolyte imbalance, particularly K^+.
- Treat symptomatically – metoclopromide 10 mg IV, orally or IM, or cyclizine 50 mg IM are good antiemetics.
- If patient is vomiting continually, keep nil by mouth and insert an NG tube.
- Treat the underlying cause, e.g. infection, pain, high calcium, gastritis.

Diarrhoea

History

- Onset of symptoms: are symptoms recent or a long-term change in bowel habit?
- What is the frequency of bowel movement?
- What colour are the patient's motions? Pale suggests malabsorption, e.g. coeliac disease; darker suggests malaena or iron use; bloody suggests colitis or ischaemia; green suggests infection.
- Associated symptoms: abdominal pain, vomiting, back pain.
- Recent hospital admission with antibiotic use
- Previous history: coeliac disease, Crohn's disease, ulcerative colitis, previous bowel surgery, AF, myocardial ischaemia.
- Drug history, allergies, any recent history of foreign travel. Recent antibiotic treatment (within 3 months).

Examination

- Vital signs, including temperature and postural blood pressure.
- Evidence of anaemia, e.g. pale conjunctivae/palmar creases.
- Abdominal examination for masses or distension.
- PR examination for masses, constipation and colour/consistency of stool. Faecal occult blood testing is invariably positive in diarrhoea and thus has limited use.

Investigations

- FBC, U+Es, glucose, LFTs, calcium, ESR, CRP and TFTs.
- Abdominal X-ray to exclude obstruction or inflammatory bowel dilatation.
- Stool cultures (×3) to exclude infection. *Clostridium difficile* toxin.
- Blood cultures if fever is present.
- Rigid sigmoidoscopy and biopsy might be required to clarify the diagnosis, especially if inflammatory bowel disease is suspected; talk to your seniors.

Differential diagnosis

- Gastroenteritis – usually viral but consider *Salmonella* and *Campylobacter* infections, along with *Clostridium difficile* infection if following recent hospital admission.
- Constipation with overflow diarrhoea.
- Drug reaction.
- Electrolyte imbalance.
- Tumour with or without obstruction.
- Upper GI bleed (blood stimulates bowel motility).
- Ulcerative colitis/Crohn's disease.
- Ischaemic colitis.

Management

- Patients with diarrhoea should be managed in a side room until infection has been excluded.

- Fluid rehydration: IV if necessary until able to drink adequate amounts.

- Correct electrolytes: especially K^+.

- Treat the underlying cause: this might require further GI investigation if symptoms persist, e.g. sigmoidoscopy, colonoscopy or barium enema.

- Give laxatives if you suspect constipation with overflow diarrhoea (this is common in older people).

- Avoid giving antidiarrhoeal agents, e.g. loperamide, unless infection and acute colitis have been excluded.

- If *Clostridium difficile* infection is suspected (i.e. diarrhoea after IV antibiotic use), send stool, for *C. difficile* toxin and culture. Commence on Metronidazole PO 400 mg tds if patient unwell.

The unconscious patient

Unconscious patients are sick patients. As with all sick patients, apply ABC first, before trying to get to the cause of the problem.

Resuscitation

- A: check the airway. Any patient with a GCS of < 9 is likely to have a threatened airway. Try and insert a Guedel airway or nasopharyngeal tube.
- B: check the breathing, listen to the chest. Check O_2 saturations and apply 100% O_2.
- C: circulation. Check pulse, BP and whether the extremities are warm or cold. Put in an IV line and take bloods for FBC, U+Es, LFTs, CRP, glucose, calcium and CK. Take arterial blood gases and send a sample for carboxyhaemoglobin if CO poisoning is a possibility.

At this point, check the BM and temperature and try to obtain a brief history from bystanders or the ambulance crew. If the BM is less than 4, give 50 mL of 50% IV dextrose followed by a dextrose infusion.

History

Look especially for a history of fits, trauma or alcohol or drug intoxication. How quickly did the person become unconscious? What was the person like before losing consciousness?

Examination

- Look for evidence of head injury.
- Feel the abdomen. Is there any evidence of liver disease?
- Do a quick neuro exam. Are the pupils pinpoint? If so, give naloxone immediately. Are the pupils reactive and equal? Is there any papilloedema?
- Note the GCS. Is one side more active than the other? Are there any shaking movements? Are the plantars upgoing? Is there neck stiffness?
- By this time, you should have enough information to attempt a diagnosis.

Diagnosis

- History of trauma, any lateralizing signs or any papilloedema: suspect intracerebral bleeding. Contact your senior immediately with a view to emergency CT brain.
- Pyrexia, rash or neck stiffness: suspect meningitis. Call your senior, take blood cultures and administer IV antibiotics according to meningitis protocol.
- Clear history of fitting: if the patient is a known epileptic and you note deterioration, observe – the patient might simply be postictal. Look for precipitants such as infection. If there is no history of epilepsy or if the patient is not improving, proceed to CT brain.
- None of the above: await bloods. High or low sodium, raised LFTs, acute renal failure, high or low glucose might explain the coma. Call your senior for advice as to how to proceed; possibilities include overdose, so send a urine sample for

toxicology, look for evidence of overdose (letter, empty bottles) and send paracetamol and salicylate levels.

- If the GCS drops by 2 or more points, or a diagnosis has not been reached, proceed to emergency CT brain. If you still have no diagnosis after CT brain, consider lumbar puncture to rule out meningitis, encephalitis or subarachnoid haemorrhage.

Other management

- Take an ECG and chest X-ray (for lung cancer, infection or aspiration). Insert a urinary catheter. If hypothermic, rewarm. Keep a slow IV running to ensure the patient does not become dehydrated; overhydration is to be avoided because it could worsen brain injury via cerebral oedema.
- Nurse in a closely monitored area, with neurological observations every half an hour to start with.

'Off the legs'

'Off the legs' is not a diagnosis; it is a label used by those who can't be bothered to think further about the presentation and its contributory factors.

History

- A full history, including a history from a relative or carer.
- Is it really 'off the legs' or is it a fall or collapse? Is it quick or slow in onset?
- Are there symptoms of infection? Are there symptoms of malignancy?
- Is there evidence of dementia? Is there evidence of depression?
- Have the drugs changed recently? Is pain the reason for immobility? Has there been a fall?

Examination

- A full examination, including mental test score and full neurological examination.
- Are there signs of infection? Are there signs of malignancy?
- Are there signs of a stroke?
- Is fluid overload (e.g. CCF) or dehydration present?
- Is cord compression present? This is easily missed and potentially reversible.
- Check for hip fracture and back pain.
- Check the feet!

Investigations

The potential range of investigations is vast. Tailor them according to your history and examination. A good basic set should include:

- FBC, U+Es, LFTs, calcium, CRP, glucose.
- TFTs if these have not been done in the last 6 months.
- Digoxin level if the patient is on digoxin.
- ECG, chest X-ray.
- X-ray anywhere with bony pain (e.g. spine, hip).
- MSU if there are urinary symptoms. Blood cultures if the patient is pyrexial.
- O_2 saturations and ABGs if $SaO_2 < 95\%$.
- A CT of the brain might be needed if there is a focal neurological deficit. Discuss this with your seniors.

Talk to your senior urgently if you suspect signs of cord compression (lower limb sensory impairment or weakness, especially – but not exclusively – if plantars are upgoing bilaterally). Hours can make the difference between walking again and being bedbound.

If you have written 'off the legs' as your final diagnosis, go back, start again, and look harder!

Diagnoses to bear in mind

- Chest infection.
- UTI.
- Stroke.
- Parkinson's disease.
- MI.
- Drug toxicity, including alcohol.
- Electrolyte disturbance (especially hypokalaemia, high or low sodium, hypercalcaemia).
- Renal failure.
- Anaemia.
- Malignancy, including cerebral metastases and cord compression.
- Hip fracture.
- Osteoarthritis of hips or knees.

Also bear in mind that the situation might have developed gradually; progressive dementia, depression, slowly worsening OA, failure of carers to cope can all masquerade under the label of 'off the legs'.

Management

This depends on what diagnoses you make – there are usually several contributory factors, so make a list:

- If the patient is dehydrated, rehydrate. Replace potassium if low; treat high calcium and derangements of sodium concentration according to cause.
- If stroke (see 'Stroke', p. 187) or MI (see 'Myocardial infarction', p. 97) are found.
- Treat underlying infection.
- Involve physiotherapy, occupational therapy and social work at an early stage; they hold the key to improving mobility and maximizing independence.
- Keep in close contact with the carers and relatives, and ensure that they are involved in the plans for discharge well before discharge occurs.

The patient with a fever

History

Look especially for:

- Cough, sputum, breathlessness or chest pain.
- Dysuria, frequency, loin pain.
- Any recent surgery or intravenous lines.
- Diarrhoea, abdominal pain.
- Foreign travel.
- Headache.
- Anyone close to the patient been unwell recently?

Examination

- Pulse, BP, repeat temperature.
- Respiratory rate, chest examination, O_2 saturations.
- Any murmurs?
- Abdominal examination, including looking at wounds and drains for infection.
- Examine current and previous line sites carefully, especially central lines.
- Examine the legs for swelling (DVT) or cellulitis; inspect ulcers carefully.
- Look for neck stiffness, photophobia and rashes.

Investigations

- FBC, U+Es, LFTs, glucose, CRP. Blood gases if unwell or low SaO_2.
- Blood cultures – take peripheral cultures, and if a central line is present, take cultures through each lumen of the line as well.
- Urine for dipstick, microscopy and culture.
- Chest X-ray.
- Swab any infected wounds or line sites. If there is a collection of pus (e.g. a boil or infected ulcer), try and collect pus for culture.
- Consider a lumbar puncture if signs of meningism are present; perform CT brain first if there are focal neurological signs or a reduced conscious level.

Management

- Paracetamol, fanning and cool sponging are good ways of reducing body temperature.
- Further treatment depends on how unwell the patient is.
- If the patient is reasonably well (i.e. pulse < 100 bpm, SBP > 100, RR < 20, not dehydrated), try and make a diagnosis before commencing antibiotic therapy. If you are happy with your diagnosis, go ahead and treat.
- If the patient is unwell, you need to get on and treat on a best-guess basis.
- Obtain IV access if not done already.

- Give fluids to rectify dehydration.
- If SBP < 100, give IV colloid, and consider a CVP line if BP still low. Call your senior.
- Insert a urinary catheter if BP is low or there is poor urine output.
- Give O_2, especially if O_2 saturations are low or the patient is acidotic.
- Give IV antibiotics. Your local guidelines will suggest which antibiotics are most appropriate for a given clinical situation. If you really have no idea where the infection is coming from, a combination such as benzylpenicillin, gentamicin and metronidazole is often suggested.

Points to note

- Not everyone with a fever has a bacterial infection. Hospital patients can also get colds and flu. Malignancy, drugs and inflammatory disorders cause fever as well, as can DVT, PE and MI. Think of these causes.
- Not everyone with a fever needs IV antibiotics. They are expensive and can cause complications. Consult your local guidelines.
- If you are not sure of the diagnosis, or if someone is unwell with fever, discuss with your senior. Incorrect use of antibiotics can obscure the diagnosis but failure to give antibiotics quickly when someone is ill can lead to a rapid death.

Fits

Ongoing fits (status epilepticus) are a medical emergency (see 'Status epilepticus', p. 108).

Resuscitation

If you are called to see someone who has had a fit, start with ABC:

- A: if the patient is drowsy, either place in the recovery position or consider a Guedel airway or nasopharyngeal tube.
- B: listen to the chest, check the respiratory rate, do the O_2 saturations. Give O_2 if $SaO_2 < 95\%$.
- C: check the patient's pulse and BP. Are the peripheries warm or cool? Obtain IV access (now – before the patient fits again!) and take bloods for FBC, U+Es, LFTs, calcium, glucose and CRP. Do a bedside Glucostix reading.

If the glucose reading is < 4, give 50 mL of 50% dextrose IV immediately.

History

If the patient is conscious – take a history:

- Does the patient remember what happened? Was there a prodrome (aura)?
- Does the patient have a history of epilepsy? Or any history of trauma, alcohol or drug binge?
- Is there any headache or neck stiffness now?
- Were there chest pains or palpitations prior to the collapse? Many suspected epileptiform collapses are in fact cardiovascular in nature.

Get a collateral history if at all possible:

- Was there any prodrome or aura? Did the patient twitch or jerk?
- Ask if the patient went rigid before the fit. Or did the patient change colour?
- How quickly did the patient recover consciousness?

Examination

- Check the temperature (although this might be raised due to the fit).
- Examine the patient for infection and for any evidence of malignancy, especially lung.
- Do a full neurological exam, looking especially for head trauma, neck stiffness, papilloedema, unilateral weakness (this can be a cause or an effect – remember Todd's palsy). Note that plantars are often upgoing after a fit; this alone is not a sign of an intracranial catastrophe.

Diagnosis

- Is it a fit, or is it a cardiovascular collapse?

Causes of fits include:

- Known epilepsy • Alcohol withdrawal • Overdose (e.g. tricyclic antidepressants)
- Stroke • Subarachnoid haemorrhage or other intracranial bleed • Meningitis
- Encephalitis • Cerebral tumours (especially lung metastases) • Low or high sodium levels • Hypoglycaemia • Hypocalcaemia, hypomagnesaemia • Acute renal failure • Acute liver failure

Other investigations

These will depend on whether the patient is known to have epilepsy.

IF THE PATIENT HAS EPILEPSY

- Check drug levels (if the patient is on antiepileptic medication).
- Look for a precipitant, e.g. infection (chest X-ray, urine culture).

IF THE PATIENT IS WITHDRAWING FROM ALCOHOL

- Check phosphate and magnesium, also INR.

IF THIS IS A FIRST FIT, NOT WITHDRAWING FROM ALCOHOL

- Chest X-ray.
- CT brain (urgent if unwell, not recovering consciousness or symptoms of an intracranial bleed, otherwise next day).
- Lumbar puncture if signs of meningism and CT brain is clear.
- Urine for toxicology if overdose suspected.

Management

- Observe closely – half-hourly neurological observations to start with.
- If another fit occurs, give diazepam and consider a phenytoin infusion.
- If blood sugar was low on arrival, give a 10% dextrose infusion.
- If withdrawing from alcohol, give IV vitamins (Pabrinex) and regular diazepam (rectally if necessary).
- Give paracetamol if fever is persistent (this can be given rectally).
- Ensure you see the sodium and creatinine results.

Points to watch

- *Never* assume that a fit is a pseudoseizure. Leave the neurology team to make this diagnosis – this is the safe way to proceed.
- White cell count is often elevated after a fit – this does not necessarily indicate infection.
- Call your senior if the GCS falls rather than rises in the hours after a fit – an urgent CT brain is required.

Overdoses

Many patients who take an overdose are not particularly unwell, but a few are very unwell. Always start your assessment with ABC.

History

If the patient is stable, take a history:

- What did the patient take? When? Was anything else taken with it?
- Why did the patient take it? What precipitated the action? Does the patient regret it? Does the patient want to die? Did the patient leave a note? Are there symptoms of depression or psychosis?
- Who else was around? A collateral history can be very useful, especially if the patient is drunk, drowsy or upset.

Don't forget to take the rest of the history as well, especially a history of previous overdoses, depression, other drugs, history of heavy alcohol intake or liver disease.

Examination

- ABC: airway, breathing – especially respiratory rate – and circulation – pulse, BP, hydration state. Is the skin hot or cold?
- Feel the abdomen for hepatomegaly; look for jaundice and asterixis.
- Do a neurological examination; pay special attention to the pupils, plantars and GCS. Do not assume that reduced consciousness is due to alcohol alone.

Investigations

This will depend on what the overdose was. FBC, U+Es, glucose, LFTs and paracetamol (perhaps salicylate) levels should be done on everyone.

Paracetamol Check the INR. Paracetamol level after at least 4 h (it is unreliable before this).

Tricyclics, SSRIs, neuroleptics, cardiovascular drugs, lithium Do an ECG.

Opioids (if drowsy), tricyclics, salicylates, unwell paracetamol overdose Do arterial blood gases.

Management

There are too many overdose scenarios to go through comprehensively here. TOXBASE and the BNF are both excellent sources of information on overdose effects and how to manage specific overdoses. Some general rules are applicable however:

- Most overdoses settle with supportive management. Close observation and rehydration often suffice.
- Emetic agents should be avoided – they do not work. Gastric lavage is almost never indicated. Activated charcoal should be given to anyone with an overdose (as long as they are able to swallow it safely and keep it down).
- Call your seniors immediately if the patient has a GCS of < 10, has signs of airway obstruction or has a low respiratory rate; intubation might be required.

- Discuss with your seniors if a patient with an overdose wishes to self-discharge. You need to assess how much of a danger to him- or herself the patient presents.

Behind every trivial, annoying, timewasting overdose case is a human being in distress – for whatever reason. Treat every person who has taken an overdose with the same courtesy and respect with which you would wish to be treated if you came into hospital with an illness. It is not your job to impose value judgements on your patients.

Ensure that all of your overdose patients receive follow-up from the local psychiatric liaison service.

Managing paracetamol overdoses (Fig. 35)

- Take a blood sample at > 4 h post-overdose for paracetamol levels.
- If the time of overdose is > 8 h, start *N*-acetylcysteine while waiting for the result.
- If the level is well below the line on the treatment graph, *N*-acetylcysteine is not required.
- If the patient is a chronic heavy drinker, has liver disease, is malnourished or is on enzyme-inducing drugs (e.g. phenytoin, carbamazepine), use the high-risk line on the graph.
- If the time of ingestion is uncertain, staggered, or the value is close to the line – treat with *N*-acetylcysteine.
- Ensure that you check the LFTs and INR on admission and at 24 h post-admission.

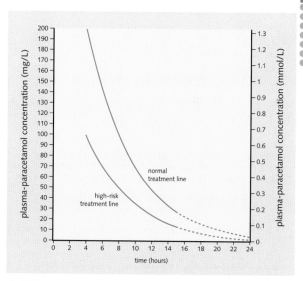

Fig. 35 Treatment thresholds for paracetamol overdose. Redrawn with permission from University of Wales College of Medicine Therapeutics and Toxicology Centre.

The swollen leg

Not everyone with a swollen leg has a DVT. Conversely, not everyone with a DVT has a swollen leg.

History

- Is the swelling new, or has it been present for years? Is it one leg or both legs?
- Has there been any injury to the leg (torn muscle, break in the skin for cellulitis)?
- Is there a history of knee arthritis or swelling in the popliteal fossa (Baker's cyst)?
- Has there been previous groin surgery (lymphoedema)?
- Are there any risk factors for DVT:
  - travel
  - previous DVT/PE
  - family history of DVT/PE
  - recent surgery or leg immobility (hospital, plaster cast)
  - any signs of malignancy
  - contraceptive pill.

Examination

- Is there a fever? Is the patient systemically unwell? Are lymph nodes palpable in the groin?
- Is the patient short of breath? Is there chest pain? (PE).
- Is there swelling of the leg? Measure the circumference of the legs 5 cm below the tibial tuberosity.
- Is there point tenderness in the calf, or bruising? Is the knee arthritic?
- Is the other leg also swollen?
- Is the leg cool, warm or hot? Is it pinkish, or is it red and angry-looking?
- Look between the toes for fungal infections and skin breaks.

Diagnosis

- If there is a pyrexia > 37.5 °C, and the leg looks hot and angry, treat as cellulitis.
- If there is unilateral swelling without looking red and angry, consider DVT as a diagnosis. Most centres now use some form of scoring system to help identify patients with DVT (e.g. Wells score (see Box)). Patients with a low clinical risk and a negative D-dimer are felt to be at low risk of DVT.

Management

FOR CELLULITIS

- Insert an IV line.
- Take blood for FBC, U+Es, glucose and CRP.
- Give IV antibiotics according to your local policy (usually benzylpenicillin + flucloxacillin).

- If fungal infection of the toes is present, treat with topical therapy, e.g. miconazole.
- Elevate the limb; cellulitis resolves more quickly this way.
- Draw a line around the extent of the erythema to monitor progression.
- Rehydrate if vomiting or dehydrated.

FOR SUSPECTED DVT

- Give SC low-molecular-weight heparin (or IV unfractionated heparin if there is risk of bleeding e.g. in post-op patients) according to your local protocol.
- Organize a duplex ultrasound scan of the lower limb veins. If clinical suspicion is low, a negative D-dimer might obviate the need for a scan because it makes the diagnosis of DVT very unlikely. However, D-dimer measurements should not be performed if the clinical suspicion of DVT is intermediate or high.
- Take blood for FBC, U+Es, LFTs, calcium and clotting. If there is no obvious precipitant, consider taking blood for a thrombophilia screen (check your local protocol – some centres wait for therapy to finish before doing this).
- If there is no obvious precipitant, go back and examine the patient for features suggestive of malignancy. Do a rectal exam, get a chest X-ray, do a PSA (men) or CA 125 (women) and consider an abdominal ultrasound.

Points to note

Not sure whether it is cellulitis or clot? Treat both and get a duplex ultrasound scan. If the duplex ultrasound scan is negative, but your clinical suspicion remains high, either:

- get a venogram or
- repeat the ultrasound scan in a week to check for progression of the clot – the scan could have missed a below-knee DVT.

Wells score to assess clinical risk of DVT	
Clinical feature	
Active malignancy	1
Recently bedridden for more than 3 days or major surgery within 4 weeks	1
Paralysis, paresis or recent plaster immobilization of lower limb extremity	1
Localized tenderness along distribution of deep venous system	1
Entire leg swollen	1
Calf swelling > 3 cm compared to asymptomatic leg	1
Pitting oedema (greater in symptomatic leg)	1
Collateral superfical veins (non-varicose)	1
Alternative diagonosis as more likely than DVT	−2

(Modified from Oudega R, et al, *Ann Intern Med* 2005;143:100–107)

Confusion

Confused patients are a common problem. Confused doctors are even more common!

- Start by checking ABC: is the patient confused because of severe hypoxia or are they about to have a respiratory arrest or profound hypotension?

History

- Ascertain whether the patient is confused – use the 10-point abbreviated mental test score.
- Take a history – the patient might be able to tell you some useful information, but check the notes and/or obtain a collateral history from relatives or nursing staff.
- Is the confusion of recent onset? The confusion assessment method (see Box) highlights those features suggestive of acute confusion (delirium) from those of more chronic cognitive impairment.
- Does the patient have sensory impairments?
- Is the patient in pain? Feverish?
- What drugs is the patient on? Are any of the drugs new?
- With what problems was the patient admitted to hospital?
- Is the patient withdrawing from alcohol?

Examination

- Is the patient breathing rapidly or very slowly? Is the patient hypoxic?
- Is the patient well perfused peripherally? Is the BP low? Is the patient dehydrated?
- Is there a fever or other signs of infection, e.g. chest infection, UTI, line infection?
- Is there pain, e.g. abdominal pain, back pain?
- Is the patient constipated? In urinary retention?
- Are there neurological signs – reduced GCS, new lateralizing signs?
- Is there a tremor, hallucinations or twitching?

Investigations

- Check the arterial blood gases if hypoxic or COPD on O_2; the patient might be retaining CO_2.
- Send for FBC, U+Es, LFTs, glucose (and perform Glusostix testing), calcium, and CRP.
- Urine for urinalysis, microscopy and culture.
- Chest X-ray if hypoxic or any clinical signs in the chest.
- ECG: myocardial infarction can present as confusion in older people.
- If the confusion is of new onset and there are new neurological signs or no obvious cause, CT brain might be required (to look for stroke, subdural haemorrhage). Discuss with your seniors.

Management

By now, you will have hopefully found several underlying causes for the confusion. Some are treatable, some might not be.

Nurse the patient in a quiet environment, avoid complete darkness at night and try and have familiar faces around, whether relatives or nursing staff. Ensure that wandering patients are watched or are unable to leave the ward area. Some patients might be better nursed at ground level to avoid falls and fractures.

- Give O_2 if hypoxic: the mask might not stay on for too long; nasal cannulas sometimes work better.
- Rehydrate and correct hypotension.
- Give paracetamol and sponging for fever. Give adequate analgesia and give laxatives for constipation.
- Treat any underlying condition, e.g. infection, urinary retention, low sodium, hypoglycaemia.
- Stop benzodiazepines and tricyclic antidepressants if at all possible.
- If the patient is agitated, a small dose of haloperidol (oral or IM) might be necessary. Do not use physical restraints on confused patients; they do more harm than good.

Points to note

- Opioids can cause confusion, but so can pain. A careful balance is necessary, and can be difficult to achieve.
- Patients with underlying cognitive impairment are at increased risk of delirium. This might occur on top of known cognitive impairment or a quite minor intercurrent illness might precipitate the delirium. Sometimes, the move into unfamiliar surroundings (i.e. hospital), coupled with sensory deprivation (night-time, lost hearing aid) is sufficient to precipitate delirium.
- Alcohol withdrawal is a common cause of hallucinations and confusion. Confusion often occurs 2–3 days after cessation of drinking and can be accompanied by tremor, fever, tachycardia and fitting (delirium tremens). Hypoglycaemia can coexist. Give regular diazepam or chlordiazepoxide, thiamine and other B-group vitamins, intravenous fluid and ensure that the patient has the opportunity to access alcohol withdrawal services if available.

Confusion assessment method (the diagnosis of delirium by CAM requires positive answers from feature 1 and 2 and either 3 or 4)

Feature 1: Acute and fluctuating course	Is there evidence of an acute change in mental status from the patient's baseline?
	Did the (abnormal) behaviour fluctuate during the day, that is, tend to come and go, or increase and decrease in severity?
Feature 2: Inattention	Did the patient have difficulty focusing attention? e.g. being easily distractible, or having difficulty keeping track of what was being said?
Feature 3: Disorganized thinking	Was the patient's thinking disorganized or incoherent, such as rambling or irrelevant conversation, unclear or illogical flow of ideas, or unpredictable switching from subject to subject?
Feature 4: Altered level of consciousness	How would you rate this patient's level of consciousness? alert (normal), vigilant (hyperalert), lethargic (drowsy, easily aroused), stupor (difficult to arouse), or coma (unarousable)

Collapses and falls

A huge range of conditions can lead to a collapse or a fall – falls especially are almost always multifactorial. 'Collapse ?cause' is not a diagnosis; go back and reconsider if this is what you end up with.

- Start with ABC: make sure that 'collapse' does not mean 'arrest'. Check that there is not profound hypoxia, bradycardia or hypotension and that the airway is not compromised, e.g. by a reduced GCS.

History

Look especially for the following:

- Was it a simple fall or trip, or was there a prodrome (vertigo, chest pain, aura, palpitations)?
- What did bystanders see? The collateral history is vital and is usually more important than what the patient can recollect (patients who lose consciousness often assume that they tripped over). Try to find out if the patient lost consciousness, if there was any shaking, what colour the patient went and how long it took for the patient to come round.
- Any previous occurrences? Any history of cardiovascular disease, epilepsy, stroke?
- Any sensory or balance impairment? Was the patient turning the head, or looking up?
- Did the patient get up quickly before collapsing?
- How much alcohol does the patient usually drink?
- Does it hurt anywhere, especially wrist, head or hip?

Examination

- Is the patient bradycardic? Do lying and standing blood pressure. Is there a murmur of aortic stenosis?
- Any signs of infection?
- Do a PR; look for melaena. Is there an abdominal aortic aneurysm?
- Do a full neurological exam; has the patient had a stroke, is the patient still drowsy, are the pupillary responses intact?
- Palpate the head, wrists and hips – look for other signs of injury.

Investigations

- Do a capillary blood glucose test.
- Insert an IV line and take blood for FBC, U+Es, glucose and CRP. Consider measuring serum troponin level at 12 hours after symptom onset.
- Send for a chest X-ray if chest signs or hypoxia are present.
- Do an ECG.
- Put the patient on a cardiac monitor if possible.

Diagnosis

By now, you should be able to decide whether the event sounds most like a:

- simple trip or fall
- cardiovascular event
- neurological event.

Management

Further investigation and management depends on the most likely cause.

- Look for evidence of a myocardial infarction on the ECG.
- If the patient is hypoxic and breathless, consider and treat for a PE.
- If neurological signs are present and there is no previous diagnosis of epilepsy, get a CT of the brain.
- Look for blood loss if a postural drop is present. Rehydrate the patient and consider why there is a postural drop. Drugs, dehydration, bleeding, autonomic dysfunction and Addison's disease are some possible causes.
- Anyone with an episode of collapse should undergo screening for myocardial infarction, with a repeat ECG a few hours after admission along with further cardiac enzymes (troponin and/or CK).
- Don't forget to X-ray the wrist, hip or any other area that is painful after a fall in which you suspect a fracture.

Once you have excluded serious and obvious pathology (which is your job on admitting the patient), other tests can be considered, e.g. Holter monitoring, carotid sinus massage, tilt-table testing, EEG. Discuss with your seniors.

People who fall regularly are at risk of breaking bones. Consider bone protection (hip protectors, calcium/vitamin D, bisphosphonates).

Falls often have many contributory causes, e.g. poor sight, poor muscle strength, poor lighting, loose flexes and wires, in addition to the causes outlined above. Involve your local physiotherapist and occupational therapist to provide a multidisciplinary assessment. Better still, refer the patient to your local falls clinic, if you have one.

Stroke

Stroke is a focal neurological deficit of sudden onset. Loss of consciousness or gradual onset of symptoms are therefore not due to stroke; look for alternative explanations.

- Start with ABC: patients with large strokes and reduced GCS, or with strokes affecting tongue and pharynx, might have airway problems. Ensure that the O_2 saturations are above 95%. Ensure that there is no hypotension; do not treat hypertension unless significant (systolic BP > 250 mmHg / diastolic BP > 140 mmHg) – then discuss with your senior.

If patients present within 3 hours of the onset of symptoms, patients should be rapidly assessed and you should discuss with your seniors whether consideration should be given to rapid imaging and thrombolyis if appropriate.

History

Take a history and corroborate it with the history from a carer or relative. Was the onset sudden? Ask about risk factors. What medicines is the patient on? Is there a history of falls? Or of heavy alcohol consumption?

Ask what the patient was like before the stroke. What could the patient do? Were there any disabilities before this stroke? Who does the patient live with?

Examination

- Perform a full neurological examination. Is there unilateral limb weakness? Is it an upper or lower motor neuron deficit (tone is often decreased in the first few hours after a stroke)?

- Is there facial weakness? Tongue deviation? Hemianopia? Dysarthria? Dysphasia?

- Is there neglect? It can be difficult to tell the difference between neglect and hemianopia. Are there cerebellar signs? Is there a sensory deficit?

- Do a 10-point mental test score and always look in the fundi.

- Examine the heart (for AF, murmurs), chest (aspiration pneumonia, lung cancer) and abdomen.

Investigations

- Do a capillary blood glucose reading, obtain IV access and take blood for FBC, U+Es, CRP, ESR and glucose (plus INR if on warfarin). If pyrexial, take blood cultures and send urine for microscopy and culture.

- Do an ECG and order a chest X-ray.

- If you suspect intracranial bleeding (severe headache, on warfarin, history of trauma or falls), discuss with your seniors regarding an urgent CT brain. Otherwise, get a CT brain within 24 h.

Management

- Ensure that TED stockings are fitted.

- Treat pyrexia with fanning and paracetamol (oral or rectal). If the blood glucose is > 11 mmol/L, start an insulin sliding scale.

- Treat fits with diazepam, or phenytoin if persistent (see 'Fits', p. 176).
- If possible, nurse on a stroke unit – patients have a better outcome.
- Unless the stroke is small and clearly does not affect the patient's ability to swallow, keep nil by mouth and start maintenance IV fluids.
- Once the acute phase is over (first 24–48 h), involve the multidisciplinary team. If there is any possibility of the swallowing reflex being compromised, keep nil by mouth until assessed by a speech therapist. Liaise with the speech therapist regarding the need for nasogastric tube feeding; do not postpone tube feeding for days on end to see if the swallow returns.

FURTHER MANAGEMENT OF ISCHAEMIC STROKE

- Start aspirin. Some centres give dipyridamole in addition to aspirin. Discuss with your team regarding ACE inhibitor therapy once the acute phase is over.

FURTHER MANAGEMENT OF HAEMORRHAGIC STROKE

- Check the FBC and clotting profile. Correct an elevated INR with vitamin K and FFP; discuss with haematology regarding platelet transfusion if platelets are $< 50 \times 10^9$/L.
- Contact the neurosurgery team for an opinion if the bleed is intracerebellar, intracerebral with mass effect, subdural or subarachnoid.

Diagnosis

Beware the following diagnoses, which can masquerade as a 'simple' stroke:

- subarachnoid haemorrhage
- subdural haemorrhage
- hypoglycaemia (check BM and give 50 mL 50% dextrose if BM < 4)
- infective endocarditis
- tumour (deficit usually occurs over a few weeks)
- fitting (Todd's palsy in the postictal phase)
- vasculitis
- encephalitis
- dural sinus thrombosis.

Points to watch

- Do not treat hypertension unless BP is > 250/140 mmHg; seek advice if the BP is this high. If BP still high after a week, treat vigorously.
- If the patient is in AF, delay starting anticoagulation for 2 weeks, unless the neurological deficit resolves completely.
- Large strokes, especially bleeds, can cause ST elevation on the ECG and result in a rise in cardiac enzymes. This is often secondary to sympathetic activation, not necessarily to a primary myocardial event.
- Keep the family well informed. Recovery from stroke is a long and difficult process for all involved. Listen to the patient and the family; be honest with them but do not take away all hope.

Headache

Headache is extremely common and most people with headache do not have a sinister underlying pathology. Anyone whose headache is bad enough to come to hospital should be taken seriously, however.

History

- Where is the pain? Unilateral or bilateral, front or back?
- Was it sudden in onset? How long has it been there?
- Is it worse lying down? Is there neck pain?
- Any associated symptoms – nausea, vomiting, watering eye, flashing lights, photophobia, blackouts, fits?
- Has the patient had similar headaches before? What medications does the patient take?
- What was the patient doing when the headache started? Is there a history of trauma?
- Ensure that you look out for signs of other systemic illness, e.g. cancer.

Examination

- Examine cardiovascular, respiratory and abdominal systems. Check breasts if the headache is insidious in onset and you suspect cerebral metastases. Check the temperature.
- Look for neck stiffness, rash or photophobia.
- Is there scalp tenderness? Temporal artery tenderness? Tenderness over the sinuses?
- Are there any focal neurological deficits? Is there any evidence of confusion?
- Check the fundi for papilloedema.

Investigations

- Check a capillary blood glucose, FBC, CRP, U+Es, LFTs and ESR.
- Order a CT brain if there is evidence of confusion, focal neurological signs or papilloedema. A sudden-onset severe headache, unlike previous headaches, could be a subarachnoid haemorrhage – an urgent CT brain is required. Remember that a negative CT brain does not rule out subarachnoid haemorrhage; lumbar puncture is required if the scan is negative.
- If there are signs of meningism, but none of the above features, do a lumbar puncture.

Diagnosis

Think of the following causes of headache:

- subarachnoid haemorrhage
- meningitis/encephalitis
- benign intracranial hypertension
- cerebral tumour (primary or metastatic)

- cerebral abscess
- skull fracture/head trauma
- subdural haematoma
- tension-type headache
- migraine
- cluster headache
- coital cephalgia
- sinusitis
- polymyalgia rheumatica/temporal arteritis
- coryza/influenza, other infections (e.g. malaria)
- low sodium
- acute glaucoma
- drugs (e.g. nitrates)
- neck pathology/injury.

Management

This depends very much on the cause of the headache. Diagnose and treat the cause.

ANALGESIA

- Start with paracetamol and add a weak opioid, e.g. codeine 30–60 mg four times a day. Headache requiring strong opioids (e.g. morphine) is unusual and often indicates serious underlying pathology.

ANTIEMETICS

- Give metoclopramide 10 mg every 8 h. Nausea often accompanies headache. A quiet environment with subdued lighting often helps, especially for migraine or meningism. Consider nursing in a side room.

Specific treatments

MIGRAINE

- Use a triptan, e.g. sumatriptan. Preparations are now available as sublingual or nasal sprays. Do not use triptans in patients with known ischaemic heart disease. Triptans are also useful for cluster headache.

PMR/TEMPORAL ARTERITIS

- Discuss with your seniors regarding commencing oral steroids. The response is usually dramatic, with cessation of symptoms within 48 h.

ACUTE GLAUCOMA

- Call an ophthalmologist as a matter of urgency. Surgery might be needed.

CEREBRAL TUMOUR

- Dexamethasone 4 mg four times a day, with a slow reducing course, can help headache. Contact the oncology team to arrange palliative radiotherapy.

Surgical presentations

Surgical presentations

191

Trauma

Assessing a trauma victim with multiple injuries can seem daunting – which injury should take priority? The American College of Surgeons devised the Advanced Trauma Life Support course in 1989 and this has become the standard in assessing trauma patients. The principles set the priorities for management and are valid regardless of the degree of injury.

You will almost never be asked to manage the care of a patient with multiple injuries but it is useful to know the fundamentals and to understand the process in which you are playing a part.

History

In the case of a multiply injured patient, taking a brief but concise history is an important part of the patient's care. Clearly, a patient suffering a minor fall is going to have very different problems from a patient involved in a road traffic accident (RTA).

Take a brief history from the patient, any witnesses and the ambulance crew. Ask three specific questions:

- What happened?
- What treatment has already been given?
- Is there any change in the patient's condition?

This, together with a history of allergies, any significant past medical history and a drug history, can be taken within minutes of the patient presenting to hospital.

Management

Once a brief history is taken, there are four phases of management:

1. Primary survey
2. Resuscitation phase
3. Secondary survey
4. Definitive care phase.

PRIMARY SURVEY

The primary survey is a check-list for the most life-threatening conditions in order of priority. It should be followed in strict order:

- Airway with cervical spine support
- Breathing and ventilation
- Circulation
- Disability: assessment of neurological status
- Exposure: complete exposure of the patient for assessment in the secondary survey

Airway If there is any question of cervical spine injury, a hard cervical collar and sandbags should be used to immobilize the spine until a fracture can be excluded. Examination of the neck and appropriate neurology should be done together with a lateral C-spine X-ray. Make sure the X-ray includes all the vertebrae down to C7 and assess their alignment.

Airway should be assessed in terms of:

- factors affecting patency, e.g. facial trauma, presence of foreign body or blood
- evidence of airway obstruction, e.g. absent breath sounds, stridor
- methods used to clear, e.g. Guedel or nasopharyngeal airway.

Breathing
- Note vital signs, i.e. respiratory rate, O_2 saturation.
- Examine the chest. Make note of any chest injury, air entry, tracheal deviation and auscultate the lung fields.

Circulation
- Note the vital signs, i.e. pulse, blood pressure, capillary return and skin colour.
- Examine the patient for any obvious cause of bleeding.
- Insert two large-bore venflons, take samples for FBC, U+Es, glucose, amylase and cross-match 6–8 units of blood. Make a note of all fluids given and any other drugs given.

Disability Conscious level can be assessed using the Glasgow Coma Scale (GCS) but on initial triaging the AVPU scale is sometimes used for speed:

- **A**lert
- Response to **V**isual stimuli
- Response to **P**ainful stimuli
- **U**nresponsive

GCS should then be noted in detail.

Resuscitation phase This takes place concurrently with primary survey; as each problem is dealt with as it is assessed, i.e. airway patency is secured before neurological deficit is assessed. When interventions such as drains, cannulas and airway support measures are being applied, take the opportunity to document treatment so far and review management decisions.

Then go back to ABC again – keep checking this because the patient's condition can change quickly.

SECONDARY SURVEY

Once the primary survey has been completed and any obviously life-threatening conditions treated, a more detailed examination of the patient can be performed. This should start at the head and neck for assessment of fractures and work down through chest, abdomen, pelvis and limbs. A thorough assessment should be made and documented from the most major pelvic fracture to the smallest tendon rupture. All will require treatment at one time or another.

The usual selection of X-rays should include chest, pelvis and lateral C-spine films, together with any other radiology suggested by the clinical findings (e.g. limb X-rays, CT brain).

All injuries and treatments should be clearly documented – use drawings. For major trauma, most hospitals will have a proforma that can be easily filled in; following this method of assessment even for minor trauma can help avoid mistakes and omissions.

DEFINITIVE CARE PHASE

Once assessments have been made, any decisions regarding the patient's further management can be taken. This often requires a multidisciplinary approach and your senior colleagues will usually make the vast majority of decisions. Ensure that all personnel involved in the management of the patient's treatment have been documented clearly. This should include both pre- and in-hospital management.

Head injury

The most important question to ask when assessing a head injury is 'what was the mechanism of injury?'.

The severity of a head injury in a motor vehicle accident compared with falling out of bed is obviously different; an injury with a blunt instrument is likely to cause a skull fracture whereas a deceleration injury can cause more diffuse neuronal damage. Equally, other systems can be affected, e.g. a moving head hitting a stationary object will cause injuries to the cervical spine and head.

History

Take a history from the patient, the ambulance crew and particularly any witnesses. Note the sequence of events:

- Did the patient trip?
- Was there loss of consciousness (LOC)? Note that the patient's version of events is a poor guide to this.
- Did LOC occur before or after the head injury?
- Is there any amnesia?
- How was the patient immediately after the injury? Orientated? Confused?
- Has there been a change in GCS?
- Are there any residual symptoms, e.g. confusion, paralysis, nausea, vomiting, photophobia?
- Is there any past medical history of note, e.g. epilepsy, syncope, arrhythmias, previous stroke or other neurology, e.g. Bell's palsy, ocular surgery?
- Is the patient taking any drugs? Make a note particularly of anticoagulants such as warfarin.
- Has the patient taken any alcohol – do not assume drowsiness and confusion in the presence of alcohol is due to intoxication; it might mask a neurological problem, e.g. subdural haematoma.
- Is there any other drug use?

Ask how the patient feels and also ask relatives or friends how the patient appears to them. This is particularly important when assessing children.

Examination

- Assess vital signs. Note GCS and patient's orientation. Remember that raised BP with bradycardia is a sign of raised intracranial pressure, albeit a late sign.
- Carefully note the size and location of any lacerations, bruises or suspected fractures. All wounds should be explored fully.
- Check ears and nose for bleeding or CSF leaks.
- Assess cranial nerves and neurology fully.
- Assess any other relevant injuries, e.g. spine dependent on mechanism of injury. Immobilize the cervical spine and exclude any injury if appropriate.

Investigations

Most minor head injuries do not require a skull X-ray. Any patient with LOC, reduced conscious level, any neurological deficit, vomiting or with a mechanism of injury that could lead to a fracture (e.g. blow with a blunt instrument) should have a skull X-ray, or more usefully, a CT of the brain.

If there is any residual neurology, reduced conscious level or signs of meningism, you should talk to your senior about organizing an urgent CT head to exclude haemorrhage. This should also be considered if the patient is over-anticoagulated.

Management

- Most minor head injuries can be managed conservatively.
- If a fracture has been excluded and the patient is well, the patient can be discharged to the care of a responsible adult with advice to return if there is worsening headache, symptoms of meningism or reduced conscious level.
- If the patient has drunk excess alcohol, strongly consider admission for neurological observation.
- Any residual neurology, GCS < 8 or a drop in GCS should have an urgent CT scan to exclude haemorrhage. Subdural and extradural haemorrhages can be drained surgically at specialist centres.
- Any patient with a GCS of 8 or less should be seen by an anaesthetist, considered for intubation and managed in a critical care area.

Claudication

Patients with leg pain on exercise should have peripheral vascular disease excluded. The differential diagnosis includes musculoskeletal causes.

History

- Calf or more rarely thigh pain on walking, especially on gradients, rapidly (within 5 min) relieved by rest.
- Ask about risk factors and associated diseases including smoking, high cholesterol, diabetes, hypertension, cerebrovascular disease and ischaemic heart disease.
- Take a full drug history, e.g. beta-blockers (including eye-drops; see 'Bradycardias', p. 164).

Examination

- Check all peripheral pulses and check for aneurysms.
- Examine both legs, even if one is unaffected. Look at the skin and examine for trophic changes, e.g. skin discoloration or ulcer formation. Is there an alternative explanation for the leg pain – look for joint pains, muscle tenderness, signs of a DVT.
- Check the ankle:brachial pressure index (ABPI): this is the ratio of systolic pressure at the ankle to that of the brachial artery. Normal is 1.0; claudication typically occurs at a ratio of < 0.7 and patients with rest pain have a ratio of 0.5 or less.
- Check for Buerger's sign: the leg is red when dependent and becomes pale on elevation.
- Examine the rest of the cardiovascular system for murmurs and signs of heart failure. Look for other smoking associated diseases, e.g. COPD.

Investigations

- Take blood for FBC, U+Es, ESR and cholesterol.
- Perform an ECG to look for underlying ischaemia.
- Doppler examination followed by angiography gives the information required regarding stenosis and distal run-off.

Diagnosis

A typical history together with Doppler or angiographic evidence of stenosed arteries clinches the diagnosis. Other diagnoses that can be confused with peripheral vascular disease include:

- muscle trauma
- myositis
- joint pains
- DVT
- diabetic neuropathy

- vasculitides, e.g. Raynaud's phenomenon
- lumbosacral radiculopathy/referred back pain.

Management

- Any underlying problem should be treated, e.g. anaemia, untreated hypertension or diabetes. Give aspirin and statin unless contraindicated.

- The patient should be strongly encouraged to stop smoking. Refer to a smoking clinic if one is available as well as an exercise clinic – both can improve exercise tolerance and may obviate the need for surgery. Consider the use of nicotine replacement patches or bupropion.

- If the patient is found to have a discrete stenosis, angioplasty can be performed; if there is more diffuse disease with good quality arteries distal to the lesion, then by-pass surgery can be attempted. Any patient with poor distal vessels will probably be managed conservatively.

Prostatism and chronic retention

History

Prostatism becomes more common with age. Ask about the following symptoms:

- Frequency: document how often in the day the patient passes urine.
- Nocturia: an important sign of severity and a symptom that often impinges on quality of life.
- Hesitancy.
- Poor stream.
- Postmicturition dribbling.
- Ask about previous episodes of retention and presence of haematuria. Is there any penile discharge, or pain on passing urine?
- Ask about any other medical problems and take a drug history.

Examination

- Examine the abdomen, checking for masses, the presence of a large bladder or signs of renal obstruction such as palpable kidneys.
- Perform a rectal examination and assess prostate size and nature – is it smooth or irregular?
- Check the cardiovascular and respiratory systems for problems such as heart failure or COPD.

Investigations

- Routine bloods including FBC, U+Es, glucose and LFTs.
- PSA – anything below 4 is usually benign; anything above 100 is usually indicative of malignancy. Anything in between is non-specific but the higher the value, the more likely malignancy becomes.
- If renal function is abnormal, organize an urgent renal ultrasound to exclude hydronephrosis.
- Urodynamic studies can be performed if there is doubt as to the diagnosis; in practice most patients will have these done in outpatients as routine.

Diagnosis

Although benign prostatic hypertrophy is the most common cause of obstructive and irritative urinary symptoms in men, consider these other diagnoses:

- urinary tract infection (can coexist with bladder outflow obstruction)
- urethral stricture
- unstable bladder (also consider neurological disease)
- sexually transmitted diseases
- bladder stone
- bladder tumour
- heart failure with or without diuretics (as a cause of nocturia).

Management

- Medical treatment of benign prostatic hypertrophy is usually with alpha-blockers or finasteride (a 5-alpha reductase inhibitor).
- Surgical intervention is usually with a TURP (trans-urethral resection of the prostate).
- If the patient has evidence of carcinoma of the prostate, treatment can be with surgery, radiotherapy or hormone manipulation, e.g. Zoladex injections. Treatment is controversial because many patients have indolent disease – watchful waiting might be as good a policy as early intervention for many patients.

Groin and scrotal lumps

History

Ask how long the lump has been present, whether it hurts, whether it moves, e.g. on coughing or lying down. Is it getting bigger?

Examination and diagnosis

Decide where the groin lump is by using the anatomical landmarks and work out a differential diagnosis (Fig. 36).

LUMP OVER THE SUPERFICIAL INGUINAL RING
- A cough impulse implies the presence of an inguinal hernia.
- Applying pressure over the internal inguinal ring will control an indirect hernia but not a direct hernia.

LUMP OVER FEMORAL TRIANGLE
- Lymph node: look for other lymph nodes or occult malignancy.
- Saphena varix: a blue vascular lump, which fills slowly. There is a palpable thrill on coughing and the lump usually reduces when the patient lies flat. Varicose veins may or may not be present.
- Femoral hernia: usually has a cough impulse. Check for reducibility (femoral hernias are usually irreducible, so exclude strangulation and obstruction).

SCROTAL LUMP
- Can you 'get above it?' If not then it is not confined to the scrotum and the diagnosis is likely to be an inguinal hernia.
- If you can get above it, is the lump separate from testis:
  - Epididymal cyst: one or more lumps behind the testis that transilluminate. Can be any size. These can be excised but can cause infertility.

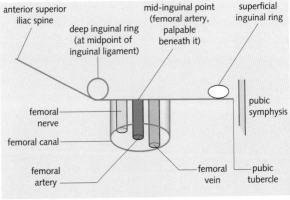

Fig. 36 The anatomical location of groin lumps.

- – Encysted hydrocoele of cord: usually a solitary lump that transilluminates and moves downwards with traction of the testis. Can be excised if symptomatic.
- – Varicocoele: does not transilluminate. Unflatteringly known as a 'bag of worms' and is marked when standing. Left-sided varicocoeles can occasionally be caused by renal cell carcinoma occluding the left renal vein.
- If the lump cannot be separated from testis:
- – Tumour: the testis is heavy and irregular, perhaps with a secondary hydrocoele. The patient will need an orchidectomy and possibly further adjunctive therapy.
- – Hydrocoele: a lump that feels cystic surrounding the testis and which transilluminates. An ultrasound is usually needed to differentiate between a solitary hydrocoele and an underlying tumour.
- – Haematocoele: similar to a hydrocoele but containing blood. Does not transilluminate and there is usually a history of trauma or drainage of a hydrocoele.

Investigations

- If in diagnostic doubt, request an ultrasound of the scrotum; this usually enables a definitive diagnosis to be made.
- If you suspect a testicular tumour, go back and examine the whole body for lymph nodes, abdominal masses, pleural effusions and chest signs. Discuss with your seniors and consider sending off blood for FBC, LFTs, calcium, U+Es, αFP and βhCG. A chest X-ray will also be required, pending staging investigations (e.g. CT) if the diagnosis is confirmed.

Ulcers

Ulcers are usually managed very well by nursing staff using a combination of dressings and topical treatments. Different types of ulcers do, however, indicate different underlying disease.

History

- How long has the ulcer been present? Is it getting bigger? Does it bleed or hurt?
- Is there a history of trauma?
- What other diseases are present? Ask about varicose veins, claudication and peripheral vascular disease. Ask about diabetes and other diseases affecting sensation. Is there a history of vasculitis, e.g. rheumatoid arthritis, or inflammatory bowel disease?
- Ask about drugs and other therapies that have been tried on the ulcer already. Is the patient allergic to any topical therapies?

Examination

- Assess the position, edge and base of all ulcers. Is there necrotic tissue? Is there slough? Is the area around the ulcer inflamed, suggesting infection?
- Assess for evidence of varicose veins, peripheral vascular disease and diabetes. Look for reduced sensation. Be aware that some ulcers are of mixed aetiology and that not all ulcers fall into classic patterns of presentation.

Diagnosis

- Punched-out squared edges suggest ischaemia as an underlying cause. They have a black, dry, tender base and can be necrotic all the way to bone. They are painful and seen in patients with diabetes and peripheral vascular disease. Check the peripheral pulses.
- Flat, sloping edges, which are soft with sloughy, oedematous and commonly infected bases, suggest pressure necrosis, neuropathic ulceration or venous ulceration. Neuropathic ulceration tends to be in the digits and pressure points (heels, buttocks, back and metatarsal heads). X-rays should be performed to exclude bony involvement.
- Venous ulceration tends to occur above the malleolar areas, especially the medial malleolus.
- Raised irregular, rolled or everted edges suggest a malignant cause for the ulcer. The ulcers tend to be fixed with bloody, infected or necrotic bases and associated lymphadenopathy. Common (sun-exposed) sites are the face and hands. Basal cell carcinoma has painless rolled edges, which are pearly white and slow growing. Treatment is by excision biopsy, deep curettage and adjunctive radiotherapy.
- Squamous cell carcinomas tend to bleed, have everted irregular edges and occur on multiple sites. These are excised with a wide margin with block dissection of affected lymph nodes. They are often sensitive to radiotherapy.
- Melanoma needs to be excluded by excision biopsy if a mole increases in size, pigmentation, begins bleeding or ulcerating, spreads or gets satellite lesions,

develops a red halo or becomes crusty. Wide excision must be carried out with lymph node resection if appropriate.

Investigations

- FBC, CRP, U+Es, glucose. Do an HbA1c if diabetic.
- If the ulcer is deep or inflamed, and overlies bone, X-ray the area to look for osteomyelitis.
- If you suspect vasculitis, do an ESR, rheumatoid factor, antinuclear antibody, ANCA and complement levels.
- ABPI: if abnormal, proceed to Doppler studies and possibly to angiography.
- If you suspect the ulcer is malignant, discuss biopsy with the dermatology team.

Management

Ulcer management is mired in superstition and a paucity of evidence, but a few key principles hold:

- Treat the underlying cause: control glucose levels in patients with diabetes, consider revascularization in arterial disease. A few venous ulcers might respond to tying off perforating veins. Vasculitic ulcers can require immunosuppressive therapy.
- Treat superadded infection if there is surrounding inflammation. Do not treat positive swab cultures without other evidence of infection; colonization of ulcers, often by resistant organisms such as *Pseudomonas* and *Staphylococcus* species, is very common.
- In the absence of arterial disease, treat venous ulcers with four-layer compression bandaging.
- Aim to relieve pressure over neuropathic ulcers with orthoses and other pressure-relieving devices.
- Keep ulcers clean and moist; avoid dressings sticking to fragile granulation tissue. There is little place for complex dressings with additives at the present time.
- Biopsy the ulcer edge if there is a suspicion of malignancy or vasculitis, or the ulcer fails to heal without a good reason.

Varicose Veins

Varicose veins are common, affecting one in three of the adult population. Most need no treatment but some cause symptoms of severe aching and itching, fewer still cause skin damage. Some people suffer ulceration as a result of their varicose veins which places an enormous burden on the health service.

The wide spectrum of disease, from cosmetic worry, concern that varicosities could cause DVT (not true) to intractable ulceration needs a varied approach.

History

Note how troublesome the veins are to the patient, if there are any problems with ulcers and take a full medical and drug history.

Examination

- Look for multiple superficial engorged veins and document any overlying skin changes.
- The level of incompetence can be estimated by using the Trendelenberg test. The leg is elevated and all the blood drained. A tourniquet is applied to the top of the leg and the patient asked to stand up. Rapid filling of the veins suggests that the level of incompetence is lower than the level of the tourniquet. The test can then be repeated at lower levels. This test has been superseded by the use of hand-held Doppler in the outpatient setting that can pinpoint the source of the venous incompetence; however, the Trendelenberg remains beloved of some examiners and is useful if the batteries fail in the Doppler machine.

Investigations

- Duplex scanning can be performed in some cases to help establish whether the saphenofemoral junction is incompetent and therefore requires tying off.

Management

Patients can be managed conservatively or surgically. Surgical management is controversial, with many differing modalities available to destroy the troublesome veins.

Interpreting blood results

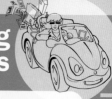

The following is a quick guide to the more common causes of haematological and biochemical derangements that you are likely to come across in everyday practice. It is not an exhaustive list, but is meant to give you a start and prompt the next wave of investigations that will be needed.

Full blood count

Low haemoglobin

Look at the old notes and look at the MCV.

MCV LOW

- Usually: iron deficiency, thalassaemia, or anaemia of chronic disease.
- Look for a source of blood loss.
- Check ferritin, iron and transferrin, depending on your local guidelines.
- If the MCV is very low for the degree of anaemia, suspect thalassaemia – ask for haemoglobin electrophoresis.

MCV NORMAL

- Anaemia of chronic disease (infection, inflammation, malignancy).
- Sideroblastic anaemia.
- Combined iron and vitamin B_{12}/folate deficiency.
- Chronic renal failure.
- Check ESR, CRP, iron stores, vitamin B_{12}, folate, blood film and renal function.

MCV RAISED

- Vitamin B_{12} and/or folate deficiency.
- Reactive to acute haemorrhage.
- Alcohol plus other cause for anaemia.
- Sideroblastic anaemia.
- Hypothyroidism.
- Check vitamin B_{12}, folate, blood film, LFTs, reticulocyte count, TFT.

Raised haemoglobin

- Polycythaemia rubra vera.
- Secondary polycythaemia (usually due to COPD, fibrotic lung disease or cyanotic heart disease).
- Dehydration.
- Check the O_2 saturations and blood gases, ask for a blood film.

Low WCC

NEUTROPENIA

- Overwhelming infection.
- Typhoid.
- Bone marrow failure (e.g. leukaemia, myelodysplasia).
- Chemotherapy.
- SLE.

LYMPHOPENIA
- Infection, especially viral and including HIV.
- SLE.
- Steroids.
- Lymphoma.
- Chemotherapy/radiotherapy.

High WCC

NEUTROPHILIA
- Infection.
- Inflammation (e.g. pancreatitis, vasculitis).
- Stress response (e.g. DKA, MI, fracture, bleeding).
- Malignancy.
- Steroids.

EOSINOPHILIA
- Parasitic infection.
- Malignancy, especially with metastases.
- Vasculitis.
- Systemic allergic disorders.

LYMPHOCYTOSIS
- Viral infection.
- TB, whooping cough, brucellosis.
- Lymphocytoid malignancy (e.g. CLL, lymphoma, Waldenstrom's macroglobulinaemia).

  Unsure as to the cause? Ask for a blood film.

Low platelets

- Artefact (due to clumping).
- Bone marrow failure (e.g. malignancy, myelodysplasia, leukaemia).
- DIC.
- Autoimmune (e.g. SLE, ITP, antiphospholipid syndrome).

High platelets

- Reactive (infection, inflammation, stress response).
- Essential thrombocytosis.

Unsure as to the cause? Ask for a blood film.
  For DIC, check the clotting, fibrinogen and D-dimers urgently.

Biochemistry

High sodium

- Almost always due to dehydration.
- Check glucose (HONK, DKA), other U+Es.
- Rehydrate.

Low sodium

Assess the patient's clinical status. If dry, this might be due to:

- Too much dextrose, not enough saline (especially postoperatively).
- Diuretics.
- Addison's disease.
- Acute renal failure.
- Salt-losing nephropathy.

If euvolaemic, this might be due to:

- Acute renal failure.
- Too much dextrose.
- SIADH.
- Liver disease.
- Diuretics.
- Salt-losing nephropathy.

If fluid overloaded, this might be due to:

- Cardiac failure.
- Too much dextrose.
- Liver disease.
- Nephrotic syndrome.

Look for diuretics and stop them if at all possible (but not if the patient is in CCF or liver failure), and examine what fluids have been given. Get a urine osmolality and urine sodium (don't get a plasma osmolality – you can calculate this: [2(Na$^+$ + K$^+$) + urea + glucose]. If Addison's disease is a possibility, talk to your team about a short Synacthen test.

Note: you cannot diagnose SIADH if the patient is on diuretics or is not euvolaemic.

High potassium

Make sure you recheck this; a common cause is a lysed sample – usually because it is several hours old. Causes include:

- Acute renal failure.
- Potassium sparing diuretics.
- ACE inhibitors.
- Addison's disease.
- Potassium supplements.

Check the drug chart and check the U+Es (see 'Acute renal failure', p. 117, for more details)

Low potassium

- Diuretics.
- Steroids.
- Salbutamol.
- Any severe illness, including MI and sepsis.
- Liver disease, especially alcoholic liver disease.
- Cardiac failure.
- Some forms of renal disease.
- Diarrhoea.

Look for the cause and replace the potassium. If the potassium is very low, the magnesium is likely to be low too – check this.

High calcium

Make sure that the calcium is corrected for the albumin level.

- Primary hyperparathyroidism.
- Malignancy (bony metastases, myeloma, paraneoplastic from lung cancer).
- Calcium supplements.
- Excess of vitamin D.
- Check the PTH – take this blood before treatment starts:
  - if the PTH is low: do a myeloma screen, chest X-ray, history and examination for cancer. A bone scan will almost certainly be needed.
  - if the PTH is normal or high: primary hyperparathyroidism is the likely diagnosis.

Low calcium

- Lack of vitamin D.
- Chronic renal failure.
- Acute pancreatitis.
- Rhabdomyolysis.
- Low magnesium levels.
- Hypoparathyroidism.

Check the U+Es and, if the history is suggestive, the amylase and CK. Check the magnesium. If no cause is found, check the PTH, alkaline phosphatase, phosphate and vitamin D levels.

High urea

- Renal failure.

If urea is disproportionately high relative to creatinine, suspect:

- Dehydration.
- GI bleed.
- Steroids.

Low urea

- Small person.
- Malnutrition.
- Liver disease.

High creatinine

- Renal failure.
- Trimethoprim.
- Eating a lot of red meat.

Low albumin

- Infection/inflammation is by far the most common cause.
- Malnutrition.
- Nephrotic syndrome.
- Liver disease.
- Protein losing enteropathy.

Check the CRP, ESR, FBC, LFTs, U+Es, urine dipstick. Do a 24-h urine collection for protein if proteinuria is present on dipstick.

Raised CRP

- Infection.
- Vasculitis.
- Malignancy.
- Pancreatitis.
- Trauma.

Raised ESR

As above. ESR raised with normal CRP can be caused by:
- SLE.
- Giant cell arteritis/polymyalgia rheumatica.
- Myeloma.
- Anaemia.

Raised CK

- Myocardial infarction.
- Falls or other mechanical damage to muscle.
- Rhabdomyolysis.
- Statins.
- Polymyositis.
- Hypothyroidism.

- IM injections.
- IM infection/haematoma.

Check the troponin level and ECG; if these are normal and the cause is unclear, check TFTs, ESR, CRP. Stop statins and see if CK falls.

Raised bilirubin

- Gallstones (in common bile duct).
- Pancreatic cancer.
- Liver metastases.
- Hepatitis (viral, chemical, drugs, autoimmune, alcohol).
- Alcoholic liver disease.

A lone raised bilirubin could be due to:

- Gilbert's disease.
- Haemolysis.

A liver ultrasound is a good place to start. For a lone raised bilirubin with no previous history of jaundice, check FBC and blood film.

Raised ALT

- Hepatitis.
- Can be due to gallstones, liver metastases.

ALT (unlike AST) is fairly specific for hepatocellular damage. Do a liver ultrasound and, if the level is > 200, a hepatitis screen.

Raised alkaline phosphatase

- Liver disease (especially obstructive lesions, metastases and primary biliary cirrhosis).
- Bone disease (metastases, Paget's disease, osteomalacia).

Try and decide from the history, examination and LFTs which is most likely. Isoenzymes (liver versus bone) can be done but are expensive and time-consuming.

- For liver disease: get a liver ultrasound, and consider autoantibodies.
- For bone disease: check calcium, vitamin D and consider a bone scan.

Arterial blood gases (ABGs)

Fig. 37 gives the ABGs for some common conditions.

CAUSES OF A METABOLIC ACIDOSIS

If the cause is unclear, do U+Es, LFTs, glucose, bicarbonate and chloride. Calculate the anion gap: $[(Na^+ + K^+) - (Cl^- + HCO_3^-)]$. Normal = 8 to 16 mmol/L.

- Causes of a high anion gap: DKA, renal failure, lactic acidosis (from liver failure, shock, systemic inflammatory response, metformin, profound hypoxia), alcoholic ketoacidosis, overdose of aspirin, methanol, ethylene glycol, tricyclic antidepressants.
- Do a salicylate level, lactate and amylase. If still in doubt, measure the serum osmolality (this will be higher than expected in methanol and ethylene glycol

ABGs for some common conditions			
Condition	pH	pCO$_2$	Bicarbonate
Metabolic acidosis	< 7.35	< 4.8	Low
Metabolic alkalosis	> 7.45	> 6.1	High
Respiratory acidosis (acute)	< 7.35	> 6.1	Normal or high
Compensated respiratory acidosis	7.35 –7.40	> 6.1	High
Respiratory alkalosis	> 7.45	< 4.8	Normal or low
Mixed metabolic and respiratory acidosis	< 7.35	> 4.8	Base excess < –6

Fig. 37 Arterial blood gases (ABGs) for some common conditions.

poisoning) and consider serum ketones. Take a urine sample for a possible drug screen later.

- Causes of a normal anion gap acidosis: usually due to excessive loss of bicarbonate, e.g. renal tubular acidosis, pancreatic fistula, ureterosigmoidostomy, diarrhoea. Can be due to failure to excrete acid (renal tubular acidosis, acetazolamide therapy, Addison's disease).

CAUSES OF A METABOLIC ALKALOSIS
Vomiting, bicarbonate excess, hypokalaemia.

CAUSES OF RESPIRATORY ACIDOSIS
This signifies failure to ventilate adequately; COPD is the most common cause. Exhaustion from pneumonia, pulmonary oedema and acute asthma also produces this picture and signifies that the patient is close to a respiratory arrest and needs ventilatory support. Neuromuscular problems (e.g. Guillain–Barré, myasthenia gravis) and mechanical problems (chest trauma, gross obesity, severe kyphoscoliosis) can also cause respiratory acidosis, as can sedative drugs, especially opioids.

CAUSES OF A RESPIRATORY ALKALOSIS

- Hypoxia (PE, asthma, infection, pneumothorax, pulmonary oedema).
- Pain, especially pleuritic or peritonitic pain.
- Aspirin overdose.
- Intracranial catastrophe, e.g. stroke, subarachnoid haemorrhage.
- Anxiety: rule out other pathology before diagnosing anxiety.

CAUSES OF A MIXED METABOLIC/RESPIRATORY ACIDOSIS

Profound hypoxia or circulatory collapse together with ventilatory failure, e.g. cardiac arrest, severe pulmonary oedema, severe pneumonia.

ECG interpretation

Interpretation of the standard 12-lead ECG usually strikes fear into most junior (and some not so junior) doctors. The fear of missing an important diagnosis means that there is a degree of nervousness when presented with one. But... look at them you must and they really aren't as scary as they first appear.

Although pattern recognition is important in making an ECG diagnosis, a systematic approach to ECG interpretation cannot be beaten – and it may allow you to make a diagnosis missed by your seniors!

A detailed chapter on ECG diagnoses is beyond the scope of this book but a basic summary is outlined here.

Patient and ECG details

Read the name, date and time on the top of the ECG. Make sure they all correlate with the patient you are dealing with. If there are a number of ECGs for a single admission, numbering them is useful, though writing anything else, e.g. diagnosis, or highlighting abnormalities is strongly discouraged.

Heart rate

The standard paper speed is 25 mm/s. Hence one small square on the ECG is equivalent to 0.04 s; one large square is 0.2 s

The quickest way to calculate the heart rate is to count the number of large squares between QRS complexes and divide into 300, e.g. if there are three large squares, the heart rate is 100 beats/min.

A heart rate of > 100 bpm is a tachycardia (Fig. 38); < 60 bpm is a bradycardia (Fig 39).

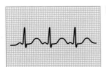

Fig. 38 Sinus tachycardia.

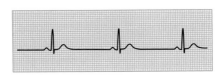

Fig. 39 Sinus bradycardia.

Heart rhythm

Is it regular or irregular?

If there is any doubt, use a piece of paper to map out three or four consecutive beats and see whether the rate is the same further along the ECG.

Regular rhythms

- P wave precedes every QRS complex with consistent PR interval is sinus rhythm.
- No discernable P wave preceding each QRS but narrow regular QRS complexes is a nodal or junctional rhythm.

Irregular rhythms

- No discernable P waves preceding each QRS complex with an irregular rate is atrial fibrillation.
- P wave preceding each QRS with consistent PR interval, the rhythm is sinus arrhythmia.
- If P waves are present but there is progressive lengthening of the PR interval ending with non-conducted P wave ('dropped beat') followed by a normally conducted P wave with a shorter PR interval, the patient is in Wenckebach's (or Mobitz type I) 2nd degree AV block.

Cardiac axis

There is nothing mysterious about working out the cardiac (or QRS) axis. It represents the net depolarization through the myocardium and is worked out using the limb leads, in particular leads I and aVF. The directions of each of these leads (the cardiac vector) are summarized in Fig. 40. By convention, the direction of lead I is 0°; and aVF points down (aV'FEET').

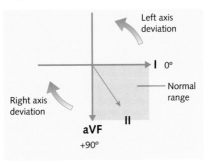

Fig. 40 The normal QRS or cardiac axis

The rules for working out the cardiac axis are as follows:

- Calculate the net deflection of each lead – e.g. in lead I, if there is a Q wave measuring three small squares and an R wave height of six small squares, the net deflection is +3. Do this for leads I and aVF.
- A net positive deflection goes in the direction of the vector; negative deflections go in the opposite direction of the vector – e.g. net deflection of +3 in I goes 3 points in the direction of I; a net deflection of −5 in aVF goes in the opposite deflection of the vector (i.e. upwards) by 5 points.
- The cardiac vector is therefore the sum of the individual vectors from I and aVF – e.g. +3 in I, −5 in aVF gives a vector of about −60° (Fig. 41). A normal axis is between 0° and +90°; anything to the left of 0° is termed left axis deviation; anything to the right of 90° is right axis deviation.

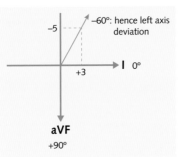

Fig. 41 Example of an abnormal QRS Axis.

P waves

Look at the P wave shape.

- Peaked P waves (P pulmonale) suggest right atrial hypertrophy – e.g. pulmonary hypertension or tricuspid stenosis (Fig. 42).

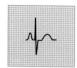

Fig. 42 Tall P wave.

- Bifid broad P waves (P mitrale) suggests left atrial hypertrophy – e.g. mitral stenosis (Fig. 43).

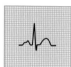

Fig. 43 Bifid P wave.

PR interval

The PR interval is measured from the beginning of the P wave to the R wave and is usually 1 large square in duration (0.2 s). A short PR interval represents rapid conduction across the AV node, usually through an accessory pathway (e.g. Wolff–Parkinson–White syndrome) (Fig. 44).

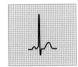

Fig. 44 Short PR interval.

A long PR interval (>1 large square) but preceding every QRS complex by the same distance is first degree AV block (Fig. 45). This is usually not significant, though it is worth checking the patient's drug history for beta-blockers or rate-limiting calcium antagonists, e.g. verapamil and diltiazem.

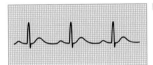

Fig. 45 First degree AV block.

A PR interval that lengthens with each consecutive QRS complex, followed by a P wave which has no QRS complex and then by a P wave with a short PR interval, is Wenckebach's (or Mobitz type I) 2nd degree AV block (Fig. 46).

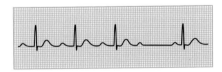

Fig. 46 Second degree AV block; Mobitz I.

If the P waves that are followed by a QRS complex have a normal PR interval, with the occasional non-conducted P wave – i.e. a P wave with no subsequent QRS complex (a 'dropped beat'), the rhythm is said to be Mobitz type II 2nd degree AV block (Fig. 47).

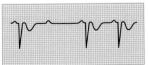

Fig. 47 Second degree AV block; Mobitz II.

If the P waves regularly fail to conduct, say every 2 or 3 beats, the patient is said to be in 2:1 (or 3:1 etc.) heart block.

If the P waves are regular (usually at a rate of about 90) and the QRS complexes are regular (heart rate about 40 bpm), but there is no association between the two, then the rhythm is complete (or 3rd degree) AV block (Fig. 48). This rhythm will need to be discussed with your seniors as will usually require cardiac pacing, and if the patient is compromised, e.g. hypotensive, will need insertion of a temporary pacing wire.

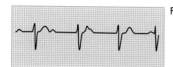

Fig. 48 Third degree AV block.

QRS complex

First, look at the width of the QRS, then the morphology.

Normal QRS duration is less than three small squares (0.12 s) and represents normal conduction through the AV node and the bundle of His.

A broad QRS complex signifies either:

1. The beat is ventricular in origin, e.g. an ectopic beat, or

2. There is a bundle branch block.

A broad QRS complex with an RSR pattern in V1 represents right bundle branch block.

A broad QRS with an 'M' pattern in lead I represents left bundle branch block (Fig. 49).

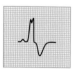

Fig. 49 Wide QRS (showing LBBB in lead 1).

The first negative deflection of a QRS complex is the Q wave. If the Q wave is > 2 mm (two small squares), it is considered pathological (Fig. 50).

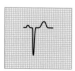

Fig. 50 Deep Q wave.

ST segments

There are basically three abnormalities seen in the ST segement:

1. ST depression – could signify cardiac ischaemia (Fig. 51).

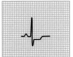

Fig. 51 ST depression.

2. ST elevation – highly suggestive of infarction (Fig. 52).

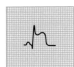

Fig. 52 ST elevation.

3. 'Saddle shaped' – concave ST segments usually seen across all the ECG, suggesting a diagnosis of pericarditis.

If there is any evidence of ST segment abnormality, particularly in the context of a patient with chest pain, seek senior advice at once.

It is important to note that ST segments are abnormal and cannot be interpreted in patients with bundle branch block, especially LBBB.

QT interval

The QT interval is usually about 0.4 s (two large squares) and is important as prolongation can lead to serious ventricular arrhythmias such as torsades de pointes. It can be prolonged for several reasons – including drugs such as amiodarone, sotalol and some anti-histamines – so a drug history is crucial if this abnormality is seen. A family history of sudden cardiac death is also important as a congenital long QT syndrome may be present.

T waves

T waves should be upright in all leads other than leads III and V1 where an inverted T wave can be a normal variant.

Tall tented T waves could represent hyperkalaemia (Fig. 53).

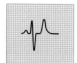

Fig. 53 Tall T wave.

T wave inversion can represent coronary ischaemia, previous infarction or electrolyte abnormality such as hypokalaemia (Fig. 54).

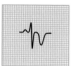

Fig. 54 T wave inversion.

Arrhythmias

Arrhythmias – be they tachyarrhythmias or bradyarrhythmias – should be treated in the context of the patient's clinical condition. Thus, vital signs – e.g. blood pressure, oxygen saturations, conscious level – should all be known before treatment is instituted. You are much more concerned about the patient with a heart rate of 140 bpm and a systolic blood pressure of 60 mmHg than you are about the patient with a heart rate of 40 bpm with a normal blood pressure eating their lunch.

Bradyarrhythmias

Any heart rate below 60 bpm is considered a bradycardia. This heart rhythm could be anything from a sinus bradycardia or atrial fibrillation with a low ventricular rate to some form of heart block as outlined above.

Treatment of a compromised patient usually requires the insertion of a temporary pacing wire and your seniors should be alerted immediately in the event.

Tachyarrhythmias

Patients with tachyarrhythmias and any evidence of haemodynamic compromise should be considered for emergency DC cardioversion.

There are broadly two types of tachyarrythmia:

1. Narrow complex (QRS duration <120 ms)
2. Broad complex (QRS duration >120 ms)

Narrow complex tachycardias are supra-ventricular (i.e. above the ventricle) in origin. If the rhythm is irregular, the likely diagnosis is that of atrial fibrillation with a fast ventricular response (Fig. 55).

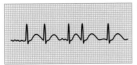

Fig. 55 Atrial fibrillation.

If the rhythm is regular with a heart rate of about 150 bpm, there is a strong likelihood that the rhythm is atrial flutter with 2:1 AV block (Fig. 56). Administration of adenosine (6–12 mg IV) can be useful in increasing the degree of AV block and reveal underlying flutter waves.

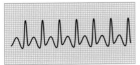

Fig. 56 Atrial flutter with 2:1 block.

If the rhythm is regular with a high rate (150–220 bpm), the likely diagnosis is a supraventricular tachycardia (either an AV nodal re-entrant tachycardia (AVNRT) (Fig. 57) or an AV re-entrant tachycardia (AVRT).

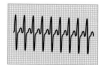

Fig. 57 AV re-entrant tachycardia.

Broad complex tachycardias are either:

- ventricular in origin (ventricular tachycardia (VT)) or
- supra-ventricular in origin but have a pre-existing or rate-related bundle branch block. An old ECG may be helpful in this group.

As a general rule, any patient with a history of ischaemic heart disease with a broad complex tachycardia should be treated as if it were VT unless proven otherwise. Call your senior.

The following are useful features to look out for that favour a diagnosis of VT over an SVT with bundle branch block:

- capture beats – normal narrow complex beats 'captured' between the broad beats of the tachycardia (Fig. 58).

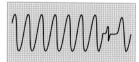

Fig. 58 Ventricular tachycardia with capture beat.

- fusion beats – similar to capture beats but the narrow QRS complex is superimposed by the broad ventricular beats.
- extreme axis deviation, usually left axis deviation.
- chest lead concordance – the chest leads V1–V6 all point the same way, i.e. all positive deflections or all predominantly negative directions.

Clinical examination

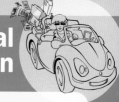

Clinical examination

Cardiovascular examination

Nail changes

- Splinter haemorrhages: infective endocarditis, trauma, vasculitis.
- Clubbing: infective endocarditis, cyanotic congenital heart disease.

Hands

- Janeway lesions: infective endocarditis.
- Osler's nodes: infective endocarditis.

Pulse

- Slow rising: aortic stenosis.
- Collapsing: aortic regurgitation.
- Bisferiens: mixed aortic valve disease.
- Alternans: severe heart failure.
- Radio-radial delay: dissecting aortic aneurysm, subclavian stenosis.
- Radio-femoral delay: dissecting aortic aneurysm, coarctation of the aorta, iliofemoral stenosis.

Blood pressure

- High: idiopathic, anxiety, pain, Cushing's syndrome, acromegaly, Conn's syndrome, renal artery stenosis, renal failure, fluid overload, phaeochromocytoma, coarctation of the aorta, porphyria.
- Low: shock states, young person, heart failure, Addison's disease, antihypertensives.
- Wide pulse pressure: aortic regurgitation, isolated systolic hypertension.
- Narrow pulse pressure: hypovolaemia, aortic stenosis.
- Malar flush: pulmonary hypertension (e.g. mitral stenosis, PPH); carcinoid syndrome.

JVP

- Elevated: right heart failure, constrictive pericarditis, large pericardial effusion, left-to-right shunting, SVC obstruction.
- Giant V waves: tricuspid regurgitation.
- Rapid Y descent: constrictive pericarditis.
- Cannon waves: ventricular tachycardia, complete heart block.

Apex beat

- Displaced: CCF, mitral regurgitation, aortic regurgitation, ipsilateral lung fibrosis or collapse; contralateral pleural effusion or tension pneumothorax.
- Tapping: mitral stenosis.

- Volume overloaded (dilatation): CCF, mitral regurgitation, aortic regurgitation.
- Pressure overloaded (hypertrophy): hypertension, aortic stenosis, HOCM.

Heart sounds (HS)

- Loud 1st HS: mitral stenosis, prosthetic valve, atrial myxoma.
- Soft 1st HS: mitral regurgitation, calcified mitral stenosis, CCF, pericardial effusion, COPD.
- Loud 2nd HS: prosthetic valve, hypertension (loud A2), pulmonary hypertension (loud P2).
- Soft 2nd HS: aortic stenosis, aortic regurgitation, CCF, pericardial effusion, COPD.
- Fixed splitting on inspiration: atrial septal defect.
- Reversed splitting on inspiration: aortic stenosis, left bundle branch block, HOCM.
- 3rd HS: normal in young patients, CCF.
- 4th HS: hypertension, HOCM.

Systolic murmur

- Ejection systolic: aortic sclerosis, high output states (flow murmur), aortic stenosis, pulmonary stenosis, coarctation of the aorta, HOCM.
- Pansystolic: mitral regurgitation, tricuspid regurgitation, VSD.
- Late systolic: mitral valve prolapse.

Diastolic murmur

- Early diastolic: aortic regurgitation, pulmonary regurgitation.
- Mid-diastolic: mitral stenosis.
- Murmur present throughout the cardiac cycle: mixed aortic or mixed mitral valve disease, patent ductus arteriosus, AV fistula.

Ankle oedema

- Bilateral: CCF, venous insufficiency, hypoalbuminaemia.
- Unilateral: DVT, cellulitis, trauma, ruptured Baker's cyst, lymphatic obstruction.

Respiratory examination

Nail changes

Clubbing: bronchial carcinoma, lung abscess, empyema, bronchiectasis (including cystic fibrosis), fibrotic lung disease.

Asterixis

Carbon dioxide retention (also renal failure, hepatic failure).

Pulse

Bounding in carbon dioxide retention.

JVP

Elevated in cor pulmonale.

Trachea

- Deviated towards areas of collapse and fibrosis (especially in the upper lobe).
- Deviated away from effusions, tension pneumothorax.

Enlarged lymph nodes

Lung cancer, head and neck cancer, lymphoma, intra-abdominal malignancy, infection.

Reduced expansion

- Unilateral: fibrosis, lobectomy/pneumonectomy, diaphragmatic paralysis, effusion, pneumothorax, consolidation, collapse.
- Bilateral: pulmonary oedema, COPD/asthma, ankylosing spondylitis and other musculoskeletal conditions.

Dullness to percussion

Collapse, consolidation, effusion, fibrosis, tumour.

Hyperresonance to percussion

Pneumothorax.

Reduced air entry

Consolidation, fibrosis, collapse, effusion, bronchoconstriction or partial occlusion of bronchus, lobectomy, pneumothorax, pulmonary oedema.

Crackles

Fibrosis, infection, bronchiectasis, pulmonary oedema.

Vocal Resonance

- Increased: consolidation, occasionally collapse, top edge of effusion.
- Decreased: effusion, pneumothorax, collapse.

Abdominal examination

Nail changes

- Koilonychia: iron deficiency.
- Leuchonychia: low albumin.
- Clubbing: inflammatory bowel disease, coeliac disease, cirrhosis, GI lymphoma.

Yellow sclera

Jaundice (haemolysis, biliary obstruction, hepatocellular damage).

Furred Tongue

Dry patient, mouth breathing.

ABDOMINAL TENDERNESS

Generalized (usually with guarding): perforated viscus, intraperitoneal bleeding.
RUQ Cholecystitis, right lower lobe pneumonia, hepatitis, rapidly enlarging liver (e.g. metastases), pyelonephritis.
LUQ Pancreatitis, splenic rupture, pyelonephritis, left lower lobe pneumonia.
Epigastric Gastritis, peptic ulcer, pancreatitis, cholecystitis, gastroenteritis.
Right flank Pyelonephritis, hepatitis, enlarging liver, cholecystitis, ureteric colic.
Left flank Pyelonephritis, diverticulitis, colitis, ureteric colic, leaking abdominal aortic aneurysm.
Umbilical Obstruction, gastroenteritis, tender abdominal aneurysm, tender lymph nodes, pancreatitis.
RIF Appendicitis, UTI, mesenteric adenitis, caecal tumour, ileitis (e.g. Crohn's disease), gastroenteritis, ovarian torsion, PID, ureteric colic.
LIF Diverticulitis, sigmoid tumour, colitis, UTI, ovarian torsion, PID, ureteric colic.
Suprapubic UTI, urinary retention, PID, gastroenteritis.
Groin Incarcerated/strangulated hernia, lymphadenopathy, muscle strain.
Scrotum Testicular torsion, epididymo-orchitis, scrotal trauma, strangulated hernia.

Abdominal masses

RUQ Hepatomegaly, colonic tumour, large kidney, enlarged gall bladder.
LUQ Splenomegaly, pancreatic pseudocyst, colonic tumour, large kidney.
Epigastric Gastric cancer, lymph nodes, colonic tumour, pancreatic pseudocyst, pancreatic tumour, divarication of the recti.
Right flank Large kidney, colonic tumour. Grossly enlarged liver.
Left flank Large kidney, colonic tumour, aortic aneurysm.
Umbilical Aortic aneurysm, lymph nodes, umbilical/paraumbilical hernia. Grossly enlarged spleen.
RIF Caecal tumour, appendix mass, Crohn's mass, ovarian mass, hernia.
LIF Sigmoid tumour, diverticular mass, ovarian mass, hernia, constipation.
Suprapubic Enlarged bladder, pregnant uterus, large fibroid.
Groin Inguinal hernia, femoral hernia, lymph nodes.
Scrotum Inguinal hernia, epidydmal cysts, testicular tumour, hydrocele, varicocele.

Causes of hepatomegaly

Note: measure the span – as chest hyperexpansion can push the liver caudally.

- Riedel's lobe.
- Malignancy (hepatocellular carcinoma, metastases).
- Right-sided heart failure.
- Hepatitis (viral, alcoholic, toxic, autoimmune).
- Early cirrhosis (liver shrinks in advanced disease).
- Fatty liver.
- Budd–Chiari syndrome.
- Biliary obstruction.
- Leukaemia, lymphoma, myeloproliferative disease.
- Liver abscess.
- Schistosomiasis.
- Amyloidosis.

Causes of splenomegaly

- Massive: CML, myelofibrosis, malaria, schistosomiasis, Gaucher's disease.
- Other: as above, plus AML, CLL, lymphoma, myeloma, portal hypertension, amyloidosis, infections (SBE, viral hepatitis, glandular fever, typhoid, TB, brucellosis), ITP, Felty's syndrome, SLE, vitamin B_{12} deficiency, thalassaemia, other haemolytic anaemias.

Causes of enlarged kidneys

The kidneys might be palpable (especially on the right) in thin individuals. Causes of enlargement are:

- polycystic kidneys
- renal tumour
- simple renal cyst
- hydronephrosis
- amyloidosis
- single functioning kidney.

Neurological examination

Cranial nerves

I   Base of skull fracture, frontal tumour, Kallman's syndrome.

II   MS, retinal pathology (e.g. diabetes), retro-orbital tumour, pituitary tumour.

III   Diabetes, vasculitis, posterior communicating artery aneurysm, base of skull tumour, midbrain stroke, syphilis.

IV   Diabetes, vasculitis, cavernous sinus disorders (tumour, thrombus, aneurysm), trauma.

V   Bulbar palsy, cerebellopontine angle tumour, cavernous sinus pathology, trauma, base-of-skull tumours, sarcoidosis, lateral medullary stroke.

VI   Diabetes, vasculitis, raised ICP, pontine stroke, MS, brainstem tumour, cavernous sinus disorders.

VII   Bell's palsy, stroke, sarcoidosis, meningoencephalitis, vasculitis, diabetes, Lyme disease, MS, parotid tumour, skull-base tumour, Guillain–Barré syndrome, Ramsay–Hunt syndrome, temporal bone infection.

VIII   Acoustic neuroma, trauma.

IX   Medullary stroke, base-of-skull tumours, trauma.

X   Medullary stroke, base-of-skull tumours, trauma, lung cancer, thyroid surgery or thyroid tumour, aortic arch aneurysm, mediastinal lymphoma, motor neuron disease.

XI   Stroke, trauma, base-of-skull tumour, bulbar palsy.

XII   Stroke, motor neuron disease, vertebral artery aneurysm, syringobulbia, MS.

Causes of cerebellar dysfunction (nystagmus, ataxia, dysdiadochokinesis, past pointing)

- Stroke.
- Encephalitis.
- MS.
- Alcohol.
- Tumour.
- Inherited cerebellar ataxias (e.g. Friedreich's).
- Paraneoplastic (e.g. lung cancer).

Causes of lower motor neuron dysfunction

- Nerve root entrapment.
- Peripheral neuropathy.
- Peripheral nerve trauma.
- Carpal tunnel syndrome.
- Motor neuron disease.

Causes of upper motor neuron dysfunction

- Stroke.
- Cerebral tumour or abscess.
- MS.
- Spinal cord compression.
- Encephalitis.
- Motor neuron disease (ALS).

Causes of absent ankle reflexes with upgoing plantars

- Vitamin B_{12} deficiency.
- Motor neuron disease.
- Syphilis (tabes dorsalis).
- Diabetes.
- Lesion at the conus medullaris.
- Friedrich's ataxia.

Causes of peripheral neuropathy – predominantly motor

- Charcot–Marie–Tooth disease.
- Guillain–Barré syndrome.
- Lead poisoning.
- Porphyria.

Causes of peripheral neuropathy – predominantly sensory

- Diabetes.
- Alcohol.
- Vasculitis.
- Amyloidosis.
- Leprosy.
- Paraneoplastic syndrome.
- Sarcoidosis.
- Vitamin B_{12} deficiency.
- Other B-group vitamin deficiency.
- Drugs (e.g. isoniazid, nitrofurantoin).
- Paraproteinaemia.

Appendices

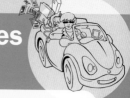

Appendices

Prescribing hints

This list is to serve only as a quick reminder during your first few days on the wards to help ease your transition into becoming a fully-fledged prescriber. There are a very large number of drugs available and the range, and latest guidance on how to use them, changes frequently. This list is not intended to be an alternative to the BNF, but rather to offer some general examples of some of the drugs you are likely to find yourself prescribing most frequently. Before prescribing any drug you are unfamiliar with, we strongly advise you to consult the BNF, especially if the patient is a child, is on other medication, is pregnant, or has liver or renal disease. Every hospital will have its own policies: remember to check these before prescribing.

Antibiotics

Amoxicillin 500 mg TDS PO. Pneumonia and UTIs
Clarithromycin 500 mg BD PO. Pneumonia, Penicillin allergy
Trimethoprim 200 mg BD PO. UTI, sometimes chest infections
Flucloxacillin 500 mg QDS PO. Skin infections (usually together with Amoxicillin); 0.5–1 g QDS IV. Severe skin infections (together with Benzyl penicillin)
Benzyl penicillin 1.2–2.4 g QDS IV. Severe skin infections
Cefuroxime 750 mg TDS IV. Severe pneumonia or UTI

Analgesia (often prn)

Paracetamol 1 g QDS PO
Co-dydramol I–II QDS PO
Co-codamol I–II QDS PO
Diclofenac 50 mg TDS PO. Good for musculoskeletal pain. Do not use with renal failure or peptic ulcer disease. Caution in elderly and in heart failure
Oramorph 5–10 mL PO
Diamorphine 2.5–5 mg IV/SC. Good for cardiac chest pain
Morphine 5–10 mg IV/SC/IM. Good for surgical or orthopaedic pain

Night sedation

Temazepam 10–20 mg PO *nocte*
Zopiclone 7.5 mg PO *nocte*
Diazepam 2–4 mg TDS PO. For severe persistent anxiety

Sedation

Haloperidol 0.5–5 mg PO/IM

Acute chest drugs

Salbutamol 2.5–5 mg nebulized QDS (can give 2-hourly)
Ipratropium bromide 250–500 µg nebulized QDS (can be mixed with salbutamol)
Prednisolone 30–60 mg PO
Hydrocortisone 100–200 mg IV (if patient cannot swallow pills or absorb oral medication)

Cardiac drugs

Aspirin 300 mg stat in acute MI or Acute Coronary Syndrome
Heparin 5000 U stat IV followed by 24 000 U/24 hours titrated to APTTR
Low-molecular-weight heparin See your local protocol for dose and frequency
Clopidogrel 300 mg stat then 75 mg per day in acute coronary syndromes with ST depression or troponin rise
Glyceryl trinitrate 50 mg in 50 mL of normal saline IV — infused at 2–10 mL/h, titrate to pain and BP
Digoxin 500 μg stat, 500 μg after 6–8 hours, then 125–250 μg per day. PO or IV in 100 mL of normal saline. For fast AF

Laxatives

Senna I-II PO *nocte*
Co-danthrusate I-II *nocte*
Magnesium hydroxide 10–20 mL PO, 1–2 times per day
Phosphate enema 1 PR *nocte*

Suggested insulin sliding scale

50 units of Actrapid in 50 mL of Normal saline.

BM >17, use 6 mL/h

BM 11–17, use 4 mL/h

BM 7–11, use 2 mL/h

BM 4–7, use 1 mL/h

BM <4, use 0.5 mL/h, with 5% dextrose infusion

Rates will require adjustment depending on how much insulin the patient usually requires, and the clinical situation (may require more if DKA or has intercurrent illness). Saline or dextrose should be run concurrently to recover and/or maintain hydration.

Glossary of abbreviations

αFP	alpha fetoprotein
βhCG	beta-human chorionic gonadotrophin
μg	microgram
A&E	Accident and Emergency
AAA	abdominal aortic aneurysm
ABC	airways, breathing, circulation
ABG	arterial blood gas
ABO	referring to the A, B and O blood groups
ABPI	ankle:brachial pressure index
ACE	angiotensin-converting enzyme
AF	atrial fibrillation
AIDS	acquired immunodeficiency syndrome
ALP	alkaline phosphatase
ALS	amyotrophic lateral sclerosis
ALT	alanine aminotransferase
AML	acute myeloblastic leukaemia
ANA	antinuclear antibody
ANCA	antineutrophil cytoplasmic antibodies
APTT	activated partial thromboplastin time
APTTr	APTT ratio
ARF	acute renal failure
AV	arteriovenous
BD	twice daily
BMA	British Medical Association
BMJ	*British Medical Journal*
BNF	*British National Formulary*
BP	blood pressure
bpm	beats per minute
Ca	calcium
CCF	congestive cardiac failure
CCU	critical care unit
CK	creatine kinase
CK-MB	creatine kinase-MB fraction
Cl	chloride
CLL	chronic lymphocytic leukaemia
cm	centimetre
CML	chronic myeloid leukaemia
CNS	central nervous system
CO	carbon monoxide
CO_2	carbon dioxide
COPD	chronic obstructive pulmonary disease
CRP	C-reactive protein
CSF	cerebrospinal fluid
CT	computed tomography
CVA	cerebrovascular accident
CVP	central venous pressure
CVS	cardiovascular system
CXR	chest X-ray
D/w	discussion with
DIC	disseminated intravascular coagulation

DKA	diabetic ketoacidosis
DVT	deep vein thrombosis
ECG	electrocardiogram
EEG	electroencephalogram
ERCP	endoscopic retrograde cholangiopancreatography
ESR	erythrocyte sedimentation rate
FBC	full blood count
FFP	fresh frozen plasma
GBM	glomerular basement membrane
GCS	Glasgow Coma Scale
GI	gastrointestinal
GMC	General Medical Council
GP	general practitioner
GTN	glyceryl trinitrate
h	hours
HbA1c	glycosylated haemoglobin
HCO_3	bicarbonate
HDU	high dependency unit
HIV	human immunodeficiency virus
HOCM	hypertrophic obstructive cardiomyopathy
HONK	hyperosmolar non-ketotic state
HPC	history of presenting complaint
HR	heart rate
HRT	hormone replacement therapy
HVS	high vaginal swab
ICP	intracranial pressure
IHD	ischaemic heart disease
IM	intramuscular
INR	international normalized ratio
ITP	idiopathic thrombocytopenic purpura
ITU	intensive care unit
IV	intravenous
IVU	intravenous urogram
JVP	jugular venous pressure
K	potassium
KCl	potassium chloride
kg	kilogram
kPa	kilopascals
KUB	kidneys, ureters, bladder
L	litre
LBBB	left bundle branch block
LDH	lactate dehydrogenase
LFT	liver function test
LIF	left iliac fossa
LMP	last menstrual period
LMWH	low-molecular-weight heparin
LOC	loss of consciousness
LUQ	left upper quadrant
LV	left ventricular
LVF	left ventricular failure
LVH	left ventricular hypertrophy
MCV	mean cell volume

Mg	magnesium
mg	milligram
MI	myocardial infarction
min	minutes
mL	millilitre
mm	millimetre
mmHg	millimetres of mercury
mOsm/L	milliosmoles per litre
MS	multiple sclerosis
MSU	midstream urine
Na	sodium
NaCl	sodium chloride
NBM	nil by mouth
NG	nasogastric
NIV	non-invasive ventilation
nocte	at night
NSAIDs	non-steroidal anti-inflammatory drugs
O_2	oxygen
OA	osteoarthritis
OD	once daily
PC	presenting complaint
PCA	patient-controlled analgesia
pCO_2	partial pressure of carbon dioxide
PCR	polymerase chain reaction
PE	pulmonary embolism
PEA	pulseless electrical activity
PEFR	peak expiratory flow rate
PID	pelvic inflammatory disease
PMR	polymyalgia rheumatica
PO	oral
pO_2	partial pressure of oxygen
PPH	primary pulmonary hypertension
PR	per rectum
PRHO	pre-registration house officer
prn	as required
PSA	prostate-specific antigen
PTH	parathyroid hormone
PU	per urethrum
PV	per vaginam
PVD	peripheral vascular disease
QDS	four times a day
RF	rheumatoid factor
RIF	right iliac fossa
RR	respiratory rate
RTA	road traffic accident
RUQ	right upper quadrant
RV	right ventricular
s	seconds
SC	subcutaneous
SaO_2	oxygen saturation
SBE	subacute bacterial endocarditis
SBP	systolic blood pressure

SHO	senior house officer
SIADH	syndrome of inappropriate antidiuretic hormone release
SK	streptokinase
SLE	systemic lupus erythematosus
SOB	short of breath
stat	immediately
STD	sexually transmitted disease
SVC	superior vena cava
SVT	supraventricular tachycardia
TB	tuberculosis
TCC	transitional cell carcinoma
TDS	three times a day
TFT	thyroid function test
tPA	tissue plasminogen activator
TTO	to take out
TURP	transurethral resection of the prostate
U	units
U+E	urea and electrolyte
UTI	urinary tract infection
V/Q scan	ventilation perfusion isotope scan
VF	ventricular fibrillation
VSD	ventricular septal defect
VT	ventricular tachycardia
VT/VF	ventricular tachycardia/ventricular fibrillation
WCC	white cell count

Please note that page references relating to non-textual content such as Figures or Tables are in *italic* print.

Normal values

Reference values may vary so check with your local laboratory

Haematology

erythrocyte sedimentation rate (ESR)	<20 mm/hour
ferritin	
female	6–110 μg/L
male	20–260 μg/L
postmenopausal	12–230 μg/L
haemoglobin	
male	13.5–17.7 g/dL
female	11.5–16.5 g/dL
iron	13–32 μmol/L
mean corpuscular volume (MCV)	80–96 fL
platelet count	150–400 $\times 10^9$/L
serum B_{12}	160–925 ng/L
serum folate	2.9–18 mg/L
white blood cell count (WBC)	4–11 $\times 10^9$/L

Coagulation

activated partial thromboplastin time (APTT)	23–31 s
prothrombin time	12–16 s

Serum biochemistry

γ-glutamyl transpeptidase	
female	7–32 U/L
male	11–58 U/L
alanine aminotransferase	4–50 U/L
albumin	35–50 g/L
alkaline phosphatase	39–117 U/L
amylase	24–125 U/L
asparate aminotransferase	12–40 U/L
bicarbonate	22–30 mmol/L
bilirubin	<17 μmol/L
c-reactive protein	<6 mg/L
calcium	2.20–2.67 mmol/L
chloride	98–106 mmol/L
creatinine	79–118 μmol/L
glucose (fasting)	4.5–5.6 mmol/L
magnesium	0.7–1.1 mmol/L
phosphate	0.8–1.5 mmol/L
potassium	3.5–5.0 mmol/L
sodium	135–146 mmol/L
urea	2.5–6.7 mmol/L